Pharmaceutical Principles
of Solid Dosage Forms

HOW TO ORDER THIS BOOK

BY PHONE: 800-233-9936 or 717-291-5609, 8AM-5PM Eastern Time

BY FAX: 717-295-4538

BY MAIL: Order Department
Technomic Publishing Company, Inc.
851 New Holland Avenue, Box 3535
Lancaster, PA 17604, U.S.A.

BY CREDIT CARD: American Express, VISA, MasterCard

PHARMACEUTICAL PRINCIPLES OF SOLID DOSAGE FORMS

J. T. Carstensen, Ph.D.

Professor of Pharmacy
University of Wisconsin
Madison, Wisconsin

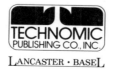

TECHNOMIC
PUBLISHING CO., INC.
LANCASTER · BASEL

Pharmaceutical Principles of Solid Dosage Forms

a **TECHNOMIC**®publication

Published in the Western Hemisphere by
Technomic Publishing Company, Inc.
851 New Holland Avenue
Box 3535
Lancaster, Pennsylvania 17604 U.S.A.

Distributed in the Rest of the World by
Technomic Publishing AG

Printed in the United States of America
10 9 8 7 6 5 4 3 2

Main entry under title:
   Pharmaceutical Principles of Solid Dosage Forms

A Technomic Publishing Company book
Bibliography: p.
Includes index p. 249

Library of Congress Card No. 92-64420
ISBN No. 0-87762-955-2

To
Cathy Gene Karr

ACKNOWLEDGEMENTS

The author is indebted for the valuable assistance rendered by the following: Dr. Z. Chowhan, Syntex; Dr. David Cornish, Sandoz; Dr. Ed Cohen, Danbury Pharmacal; Dr. J. Czeisler, Berlex; Dr. Carolyn Ertell, Rhône-Poulenc; Miriam Franchini, The University of Wisconsin; Dr. C. Kumkumian, FDA; Professor LiWanPo, Queen's College, Belfast, N. Ireland; Dr. Gene McGonigle, Schering; Dr. D. Monkhouse, Smith-Beecham; Professor Francis Puisieux, Université de Paris-Sud, France; Professor C. Rhodes, University of Rhode Island; Dr. Ed Shinal, American Cyanamid Co.; and Dorothy Dolfini, Smith-Beecham.

The following text is reading material used in conjunction with a lecture series on solid dosage forms.

A modified FDA nomenclature will be used as much as possible throughout this text. *Drug substance* will refer to the bulk drug, *drug product* to the compounded drug not in its final container. The word *final drug product* will be employed for the compounded drug in its final container.

DEVELOPMENT OF A NEW PRODUCT

The development of a new drug product starts with the discovery process, i.e., a team of scientists, most often an organic (medicinal) chemist and a pharmacologist, will (1) synthesize a new molecular entity, and (2) test it in some animal species, showing that it is pharmacologically active. (Alternate testing methods are being developed in many companies to avoid the use of animals for this and other phases.)

A small-scale batch (often a laboratory batch made by the organic chemist) will be made, and from this the following activities will result:

(1) Initial toxicity testing

(2) Analytical research

(3) Preformulation

These activities will ascertain that the drug can safely be used in initial clinical testing (Phases I and II), that it can be assayed for, and that it can be formulated into entities that would be stable, at least during the period of clinical testing (and further toxicity testing). This material is submitted to the FDA in the form of an *Investigational New Drug* (IND). The approval of this allows the company to start clinical trials.

PHASE I CLINICAL OR HUMAN PHARMACOLOGY

It should be recalled that at this point in time it is not known what the optimal amount of drug is. It may be known that x mg of drug per kg is needed in a dog, but this never translates proportionally to a human. The first series of tests are therefore prepared in a series of strengths, e.g., from 5 to 200 mg of drug.

During this period of time injections are also given, and blood levels determined, so that the bioavailability of the drug can be determined.

Administration of a solution and of a tablet are also carried out, and in this fashion it is possible to assess the areas under the curves of the tablet and the solution. It is assumed that a tablet cannot give better bioavailability than a solution, and the ratio of the area under the tablet curve to that under the solution is denoted the *formulation efficiency*.

In Phase I and Phase II clinical trials, the dosage level and side effects are determined, and are followed by Phase III clinical trials.

PHASE III CLINICAL TRIALS

Here large population groups are subjected, usually, to double-blind studies, i.e., a group of volunteer patients are treated with either placebo or active drug. (Double-blind implies that the clinician also does not know which is placebo and which is active drug.) The protocol for such studies has been worked out on a statistical basis so that it can be judged whether effects of the drug product are significantly different from those of the placebo group. Some effects (e.g., a common headache) are difficult to study, and one talks about a "high placebo effect," i.e., many patients receiving a placebo may experience a disappearance of the headache.

Once these trials are finished, the clinical findings will be evaluated statistically, and form the basis for the label claim in the insert. The data are accumulated in the New Drug Application (NDA) which is submitted to the FDA.

In this document will also be the recommended formula. A semi-full-scale batch of the product must have been made at the time of the NDA submission.

The NDA must contain stability data of the product, and detailed manufacturing instructions.

The FDA usually (where possible) requires a blood level curve and a pharmacokinetic profile of the drug substance, as well as a biopharmaceutical profile of the drug product. *In vitro* correlation (for lack of a better word) is usually attempted as well (e.g., in the form of a dissolution test).

This can be used for formula development (which formula releases the drug the most rapidly, etc.) and for quality control, as shall be discussed shortly.

SCALE-UP PHASES IN PRODUCT DEVELOPMENT

There are two aspects to scale-up during the product development process:

(1) The drug substance itself is first produced in the laboratory, then in so-called kilo-labs, where intermediate-size quantities are made. This will allow the engineering section to study the synthesis and evaluate how it can be best manufactured in large scale. In Phase III, the requirements of drug are much higher, and the material is now made in full-scale synthesis equipment. These changes can greatly affect the *physical characteristics* of the drug substance, e.g., the particle size distribution, the crystal habit, or even the crystal form, as shall be discussed later. There are hence changes in the product as the development process occurs.

(2) The drug product is first produced in small-scale equipment (e.g., a single punch, an eccentric machine), then later on slower rotary machines, and finally on high-speed machines. Compounded material may work well on single punch machines, but not on high-speed equipment. Characteristics such as powder flow and particle size distributions are therefore of great importance, and it is important to know what aspect of the compounded or un-compounded drug substance affects these parameters.

SIMILARITY PRINCIPLES IN THE CLINICAL TO MANUFACTURING TRANSITION

For the patient to be assured that the product he/she buys in the pharmacy will have the effect claimed, it is important to realize that each person is an individual in a large population, and that the company has tested the product in a subpopulation (albeit often quite large). Hence if a product does not have the desired effect it could be because the patient falls outside the test population limits, or it could be because the batch of drug product the patient is using differs from that used in the clinical trials. To ascertain with the largest probability possible that it is not the latter case, a production-scale (not size) batch is usually made before the submittal to the NDA, and a *bioequivalence test* is performed between that batch and a clinical batch that was used to establish blood levels.

In vitro tests are developed which attempt to show that the two batches are *in vitro* equivalent, and these *in vitro* tests are then carried out on each batch to guarantee to the public that there is equivalence between the original clinical batches, on which claims were based, and the manufactured batches, from which purchases are made.

The fallacy of this argument is, of course, that the *in vitro* test may not be all-encompassing, and that it might be possible to produce a batch of material that passed the *in vitro* test, but was not equivalent to the original batch. Such cases do occur, but in general a great deal of conscientious work is extended toward assuring that the *in vitro* test will reject a "bad" batch and accept a "good" batch. These *in vitro* tests are usually dissolution tests.

PLAN OF THE TEXT

The text to follow is planned in the following fashion: first, some biopharmaceutical principles are overviewed. Next the pharmaceutical operations are overviewed, since it is easier to put emphasis on the basic properties afterwards, since their effect on the macro-operation can then be alluded to. Following this, macro-attributes (dissolution, stability, and bioavailability) will be dealt with. Finally, the physics and chemistry of solids will be discussed on the semi-micro and micro levels, with referencing to the macro-phenomena and the task of the development pharmacist, the analytical chemist, and the production pharmacist. The book is particularly geared to that particular audience and, of course, to students and educators of pharmacy.

CHAPTER 1

Absorption Attributes of a Dosage Form

It is obvious that a dosage form must contain a drug that is effective, in some manner, in treating some condition or disease state. Hence, in the development of drugs, there is a pharmacological effort in the original screening of the compounds.

Finding that the drug substance is effective against some condition, disease, and/or microorganism does not, however, guarantee a marketable product or one that may be of use. It will be assumed in the following that toxicity is such that the drug substance is marketable from that point of view (although chronic toxicity often leads to the discontinuation of a drug substance as a viable, marketable item).

If, strictly *in vitro*, a drug substance is effective, is it effective if applied to an *in vivo* situation? To answer such questions, animal tests are usually carried out, and the problem of absorption is addressed.

1.1 PHARMACOKINETICS. ABSORPTION OF THE DRUG SUBSTANCE

If a solution of a substance is injected into man or animal, then blood samples can be taken at set intervals and the concentration of drug substance determined, provided a blood/drug assay exists. Hence a certain analytical effort is necessary before pharmacokinetic studies can be carried out.

A typical set of data are shown in Table 1.1. These data are plotted in Figure 1.1.

A deeper discussion of pharmacokinetic principles will not be undertaken in this text. Suffice it to say that a very simple model, the so-called

1

TABLE 1.1 Blood Level Data after Administration of 300 mg of a Drug Substance Intravenously.

Time (Hours)	Blood Level (μg/mL)	ln [B]
1	54.3	3.995
2	49.1	3.894
3	44.4	3.793
4	40.2	3.694
5	36.4	3.595
12	18.1	2.896
18	9.0	2.293
24	5.4	1.957

one-compartment model, assumes that when a drug substance is given by intravenous route to man or animal, the drug will immediately distribute in a so-called volume of distribution (V), and then disappear by way of either metabolism (k_m) or excretion (k_e).

This means that the elimination will occur by a first order process:

$$dB/dt = -k_e B - k_m B = -kB \qquad (1.1)$$

or

$$\ln [B] = \ln [B_o] - kt \qquad (1.2)$$

where B is blood level at time t and where

$$k = k_e + k_m \qquad (1.3)$$

Equation (1.2) states that when the logarithm of the blood level is plotted versus time, then a straight line results, and the y-intersect is the initial blood concentration; since this cannot be measured, it is obtained by extrapolation. The example shown in Figure 1.1 is treated by Equation (1.2) in Figure 1.2.

It is seen that the intercept is ln $[B_o] = 4.1048$ so that

$$[B_o] = \exp(4.1048) = 60 \ \mu g/mL = 60 \ mg/L \qquad (1.4)$$

If the dose given is D_i mg, and if the initial blood level is B_o mg/L then it follows that

$$D_i/V = B_o \qquad (1.5)$$

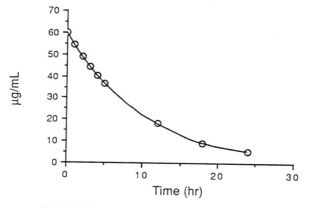

FIGURE 1.1. *Blood level data from Table 1.1.*

Hence, in the above example, where $D = 300$ mg (Table 1.1):

$$300/V = 60 \quad \text{i.e.,} \quad V = 5 \text{ liters} \tag{1.6}$$

so that the distribution volume is 5 liters.

It is also seen that the elimination rate constant, k, is

$$k = 0.1 \text{ hr}^{-1} \tag{1.7}$$

The so-called half-life, $t_{0.5}$, is an often-used parameter. This is the length of time it takes for a concentration to drop to one-half its value. In Figure 1.1

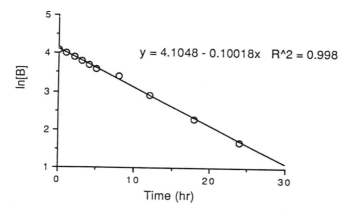

$$y = 4.1048 - 0.10018x \quad R^2 = 0.998$$

FIGURE 1.2. *Data from Figure 1.1 treated by Equation (1.2).*

the original concentration is 60 mg/L, and the abscissa corresponding to 30 mg/L is read graphically to be about 7 hours.

The half-life is given, for instance, as the length of time it takes for the concentration to drop to $B_o/2$. Inserting this in Equation (1.2) in the form:

$$\ln [B/B_o] = -kt \tag{1.8}$$

gives:

$$\ln [1/2] = -0.693 = -kt_{0.5} \tag{1.9}$$

In the data in Figure 1.2 it is seen that

$$t_{0.5} = 0.693/k = 0.693/0.1 = 6.93 \text{ hours} \tag{1.10}$$

i.e., close to that read graphically.

The antilogarithmic form of Equation (1.2) is:

$$B = B_o \exp(-kt) \tag{1.11}$$

The area under the curve, A_i, is:

$$A_i = \int_o^\infty [B_o \exp(-kt)]dt = B_o/k \tag{1.12}$$

In the above case, the area under the IV blood level curve is:

$$A = 60/0.1 = 600 \text{ mg-hour/L} \tag{1.13}$$

1.2 ORAL ABSORPTION. FRACTION ABSORBED

If the drug substance just discussed were given orally in a dose of D_o, then the blood level data could have the appearance demonstrated in Table 1.2.

B plotted versus t is shown in Figure 1.3.

It is assumed that absorption occurs during a certain period of time (the absorption or biological window), and that it ceases (or drastically reduces) thereafter. Once this point is reached, drug substance, in a simple model, is no longer absorbed and is eliminated, and hence the profile after the absorption window, t^*, should be the same as in the case of the IV administra-

TABLE 1.2 Blood Level Data after Oral
Administration of 1 Gram of Drug Substance
in Aqueous Solution.

Time (Hours)	Blood Level (mg/L)	ln [B]
1	20	2.996
2	30	3.401
3	35	3.555
4	37.5	3.624
5	38.75	3.657
6	39	3.664
7	38.75	3.657*
8	35	3.555*
12	23.5	3.157*
18	12.9	2.557*
24	7.08	1.957*

*Post-absorptive.

tion. It is noted that the last figures (asterisked) in Table 1.2 are logarithmic in time, and this is shown in Figure 1.4, and compared with the IV data. Hence the absorption window can, in many cases, be determined as the point where the data become a first order decay.

If the asterisked points in Table 1.2 and the logarithmic data from Table 1.1 are plotted, then it is seen that the elimination rate constant obtained from both are the same. This is shown in Figure 1.5.

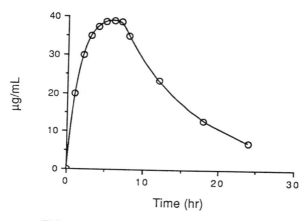

FIGURE 1.3. *Blood level data from Table 1.2.*

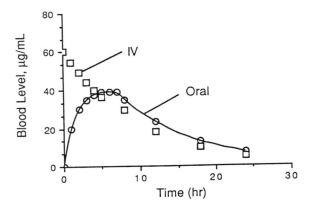

FIGURE 1.4. *Data from Tables 1.1 and 1.2.*

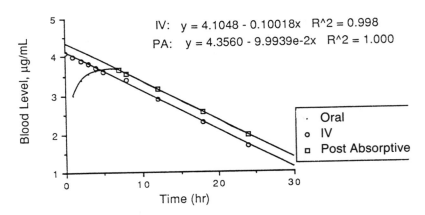

IV: y = 4.1048 - 0.10018x   R^2 = 0.998
PA: y = 4.3560 - 9.9939e-2x   R^2 = 1.000

- Oral
o IV
□ Post Absorptive

FIGURE 1.5. *Logarithmic data from Tables 1.1 and 1.2.*

The area under the blood level curve is an indicator of how much of the drug has been absorbed. By definition, the fraction of the drug absorbed by the oral route is the ratio of the area under the oral curve (A_o) to that under the IV curve (A_i) if the doses are the same.

Assuming linear dose response, in the above case, the fraction absorbed would be calculated as follows: If the area under the curve in Figure 1.3 is 550 mg-hours/L, then it would have been $0.3 \times 550 = 165$ mg-hours/L had the dose been only $D_i/D_o = 0.3/1.0 = 0.3$ g. This area, hence, is

$$\text{Adjusted area} = A_o^* = A_o \, [D_i/D_o] \tag{1.14}$$

Hence the bioavailability is:

$$Q = A_o^*/A_i = A_o D_i/[A_i D_o] \tag{1.15}$$

or

$$Q = A_o^*/A_i = 165/600 = 0.24 = 24\%$$

The problem of how to obtain areas in the case of oral absorption exists, as shown in Figure 1.6.

The best process is to realize that the absorption curve is of the type:

$$[B] = A \, \exp(-at) - G \, \exp(-gt) \tag{1.16}$$

where a is an elimination rate constant, and g is an absorption rate constant. The curve can be "feathered," i.e., at high t values the last term disappears

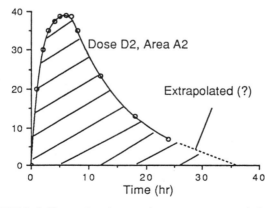

FIGURE 1.6. *Uncertainty in area determination in oral absorption.*

and the plot becomes logarithmic in time, as is, for instance, the case in Figure 1.5. Once A and a are known from this plot, then a plot of $\ln \{[B] - A \exp(-at)\}$ versus time will give $-g$ as the slope, and $\ln [G]$ as the intercept, i.e.

$$\ln \{A \exp(-at) - [B]\} = -gt + \ln [G] \qquad (1.17)$$

In general g is considerably larger than a, otherwise there would be no detectable blood levels.

The maximum in the curve occurs when

$$d[B]/dt = 0 = -(A/a) \exp(-at^*) + (G/g) \exp(-gt^*) \quad (1.18)$$

Integration of Equation (1.16) from zero to infinity gives the area under the curve, but it is realized that errors in the parameters may cause errors in this estimate as well.

1.3 FORMULATION EFFICIENCY

The oral dosage forms are usually less bioavailable than solutions. If it is assumed that the best one can obtain, bioavailability-wise, is a solution, then the formulation efficiency of a tablet or a capsule, F, is the area under the solid dosage form, A_{solid}, versus that of a solution, $A_{solution}$, i.e.

$$F = A_{solid}/A_{solution} \qquad (1.19)$$

If, for instance, in the above example, 1 gram of solid had been administered, and the area under the blood level curve was 100, then

$$F = 100/165 = 0.6 = 60\%$$

1.4 *IN VITRO* TO *IN VIVO* CORRELATION

Both in development and in the concept of quality control, there is a tacit assumption that there is a dissolution method which, in some shape, manner, or form, relates to the biological absorption of the drug substance. For initial formulation work, it is most often assumed that the faster the dissolution, the more readily will the drug be absorbed.

This, however, is not necessarily so. If it is assumed that what has been dissolved in the biological window is also absorbed, then two dosage forms could allow the drug to dissolve sufficiently rapidly to be all dissolved prior to t^*, yet have different dissolution curves. One could, for instance, give total dissolution in $t^*/2$ hours, the other in 0.75 t^* hours. The t_{max} would probably be different for the two preparations, but only slightly so, and the areas would be the same. But below a critical dissolution rate, the amount (percent) absorbed will change.

There have been cases in literature where dissolution rates have been drastically different, and bioavailabilities have also been drastically different. The dissolution rates are given, grossly, by the Noyes-Whitney equation, which states that—denoting by M the mass of a solid not dissolved at time t (of a solid in contact with a liquid)—the dissolution rate is given by:

$$dM/dt = -k'A^*(S - C) \qquad (1.20)$$

where A^* is the surface area of the drug substance, S is its saturation concentration, and C is the concentration at time t.

It is apparent therefore, that surface areas, A^* (cm²), intrinsic dissolution rate constants, k' (cm/sec), and saturation concentrations, S, are properties of great importance in solid pharmaceutics. These will all be discussed in the following.

1.5 THE INTRINSIC DISSOLUTION RATE CONSTANT

There was, in the 1950s and 1960s, a great deal of discussion about the intrinsic dissolution rate constant, k'. A so-called film theory was developed, and to determine k', a so-called plate method of dissolution was developed [1]. The method simply consisted of making a tablet in a die, and rotating this at a given speed (rpm) in a dissolution medium.

Many authors would give the dissolution rate constant in units of mg/cm³ per min, but it should be recalled that, dimensionally, k' is in cm/sec. It should also be noted that k' is a function of rotational speed [2,3] and, hence, is not an actual constant. The flux in a rotating disk is actually given by Levich's equation [4]:

$$\text{Levich's equation: } (1/A^*)dM/dt = qD^{2/3}\omega^{1/2}\nu^{-1/6}S \qquad (1.21)$$

where q is a constant with value of 0.62, ω is rotational speed, D is diffusion coefficient, and ν is kinematic viscosity.

Actual dissolution of powders in dissolution apparatuses (Figure 1.7), as shall be seen in the following, usually follows a cube root equation giving

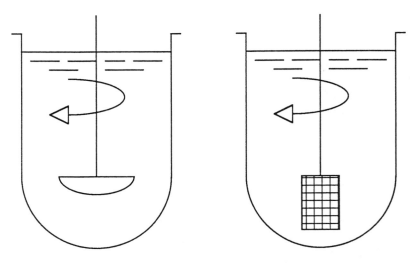

FIGURE 1.7. *USP Dissolution Apparatuses II (left) and I (right).*

rise to the type of dissolution curve shown in shape A in Figure 1.8. Tablets usually first have to disintegrate and give the type of curve shown in shape B in Figure 1.8.

1.6 DISSOLUTION TESTING

Dissolution is usually determined in one of the USP dissolution apparatuses. The principles of these are shown in Figure 1.7.

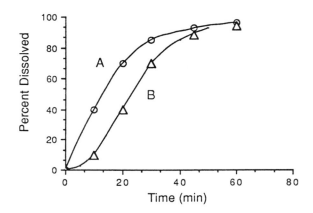

FIGURE 1.8. *Dissolution plots. A: without lag time, B: with lag time.*

The dissolution temperature is 37°C, and the rotational speed can be 50, 100, or 150 rpm. However, the FDA usually insists on 50 rpm, since this speed most often is more likely to discriminate between performances of different formulations. Again, it is assumed that the more rapidly dissolving formula will be the more bioavailable.

Dissolution media can be water, N/10 HCl, pH 7 buffer, but most often water is preferred if possible. The dissolution volume is 900 mL in the standard setup, and the medium should be chosen so that all the drug substance can be dissolved in this volume. For poorly soluble substances, solvents (ethanol) or surfactants are often resorted to. A volume larger than 900 mL can be obtained by using a different (2-liter) vessel.

The important aspect is that the dissolution test has been performed on a clinical batch, and it has been shown that clinically active batches have the specified dissolution curve. It is desirable, as well, if it can be demonstrated that dissolution curves deviating substantially (e.g., by more than 20%) from the one selected do not give adequate clinical responses. It shall be shown later that such plots are S-shaped [5] or, otherwise (if the disintegration time is short), cube root plots [6]. Such plots are shown in Figure 1.8. Once in production, however, the USP calls for a one-point method, most often a lower limit of 75% dissolved after 30 minutes.

For sustained release products there are usually three or four test points (one and four hours usually being among the times specified).

Equation (1.20) predicts that dissolution should increase with increasing solubility. One might ask, how can one increase the solubility of a compound? As mentioned, dissolution media can be manipulated to this end, but what biopharmaceutical meaning does that have? With media manipulation, dissolution testing only serves as a type of quality control of manufactured batches, and, as mentioned, to some degree assures the consumer that what he/she takes is a reasonable facsimile of what was tested in the clinic.

But in reality the solubility of a compound is also a function of the morphology of a compound, an aspect that will be discussed in later chapters. Suffice it here to say that morphology (in reality solubility) is of importance biopharmaceutically. Figure 1.9 shows a graph constructed from data published by Aguiar et al. [7] which speaks for itself.

1.7 ABBREVIATED NEW DRUG APPLICATIONS AND BIOBATCHES

In a development program, there comes a point in time when large batches have to be made. These must be made in the same equipment as that suggested in the New Drug Application for future production, and the batch size must be no smaller than one-tenth of the batch size suggested for production.

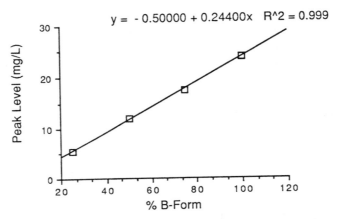

FIGURE 1.9. *Blood level as a function of solubility. Graph constructed from data published by Aguiar et al. [7].*

Bioequivalence tests are carried out between clinical batches and these so-called biobatches. The blood levels should not differ significantly, and this is to be interpreted as follows: The protocol should be made so that a 25% difference in bioavailability should be detectable with the prevailing precision. If the test has this power, and the data fail to show a difference between clinical and biobatch, then they are deemed bioequivalent.

In an ANDA, the generic company compares its product with the innovator's product by the same criteria.

The dissolution test becomes a quality control test once the product is in production, in that it, in a way, assures the public that the product sold is "equivalent" to what was tested in the clinic.

1.8 REFERENCES

1. Wood, J. H., J. E. Syarto and H. Letterman. 1965. *J. Pharm. Sci.*, 54:1068.
2. Carstensen, J. T. and K. Dhupar. 1976. *J. Pharm. Sci.*, 65:1634.
3. Carstensen, J. T., T. Y. Lay and V. K. Prasad. 1978. *J. Pharm. Sci.*, 67:1303.
4. Levich, V. G. 1962. *Physicochemical Hydrodynamics, Vol. 1.* Englewood Cliffs, New Jersey: Prentice-Hall, p. 342.
5. Carstensen, J. T., J. L. Wright, K. W. Blessel and J. Sheridan. 1978. *J. Pharm. Sci.*, 67:1, 48.
6. Hixson, A. and J. Crowell. 1931. *Ind. Eng. Chem.*, 23:923.
7. Aguiar, A. J., J. Krc, Jr., A. W. Kinkel and J. C. Samyn. 1967. *J. Pharm. Sci.*, 56:847.

1.9 PROBLEMS (CHAPTER 1)*

(1) The following is a set of data obtained from a plate method of dissolution of a drug. The disk has 1 cm^2 cross section and the solubility of
the drug is 100 mg/mL. The rotational speed is 50 rpm. The volume is
900 mL. Calculate the apparent dissolution rate constant, k', in units
of cm/min.

Time (min)	10	20
mg dissolved	10	15

(2) If the rotational speed had been 100 rpm, what would the expected rate
constant have been?

CHAPTER 2

Powder Dosage Forms, Densities and Blending

The solid dosage forms are subdivided, in order of ascending complexity, as pure drug substances, powders, hard shell capsules, uncoated tablets, film-coated tablets, and sugar-coated tablets. Soft shell capsules are essentially a subdivision of solution or suspension dosage forms, but will also be treated shortly here.

2.1 DRUG SUBSTANCE PER SE

It is possible to dispense a drug substance as-is, and in earlier times this was quite common. In the 1930s in Europe, for instance, aspirin was often prescribed as a cachet.

In this case the accuracy of dosing is the accuracy of the amount of powder in the cachet, and of the drug content of the pure drug substance. Since this is not a usual dosage form nowadays, it will not be covered further.

There are other types of products of a pseudo-pharmaceutical nature that are "one-component" systems, e.g., Citrucel and Metamucil. These are sold in bottles, and dispensed by a teaspoon. Since these products are not drugs in the strictest sense, the accuracy and precision of fill is not all that important. For instance the label will not say that one dose provides so and so many mg of fibre.

Questions such as these are still a concern of the FDA, as witnessed by the recent surge of corrective actions (the word "fresh" on orange juice, for instance) that the agency has initiated.

There are factors other than the size of a spoon (teaspoon: theoretically 5 mL, tablespoon: theoretically 15 mL), that play a part in taking a heaping

15

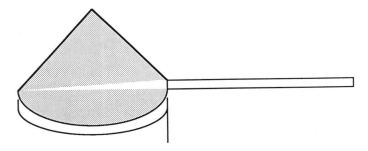

FIGURE 2.1. *Heaping teaspoon.*

spoonful (see Figure 2.1). The height of the cone in the heap is of importance.

This is best measured by the so-called angle of repose [1–6], α, which is of importance in other pharmaceutical aspects.

Particles attract one another (much like the planets attract one another). The force, c, is called the cohesive force and is proportional to the diameter [7–10] of the particle:

$$c = \beta d \qquad (2.1)$$

where β is a proportionality constant that can be determined experimentally. But the cohesive stress, i.e., the force per surface area, is smaller the larger the particle is (see Figure 2.2).

Cross-sectional area A

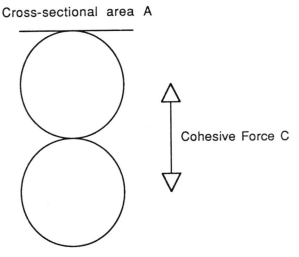

Cohesive Force C

FIGURE 2.2. *Force between two particles of diameter d.*

This can be seen by the following argument: The force per area is the cohesive stress. This, between two particles, would be c/A, where A is the cross-sectional area of the sphere (i.e., $\pi d^2/4$) and the cohesive stress, C (force/area, Pascal) is therefore:

$$C = \beta d/(\pi d^2/4) = \phi/d \qquad (2.2)$$

where $\phi = 4\beta/\pi$ is a constant. This d-dependence applies to the repose angle too [1,11–14].

In other words, the finer the particles are, the larger the cohesive stress. This is the reason that fine particles in containers (e.g., powdered sugar) have a tendency to lump together, whereas larger particles (e.g., granulated sugar) do not.

The problems connected with cohesion are often severe pharmaceutical problems, both in producing and in maintaining the quality of a pharmaceutical product.

An old-fashioned way of assessing the cohesive stress is by way of the so-called angle of repose. This is actually the angle of the heap in a heaping teaspoon. At a later point, when the problems of blending are discussed, a measurement technique for the repose angle will be discussed.

2.2 POWDERS

It is rare that a drug can be dispensed as-is. Most often convenience and marketing considerations necessitate that the substance be diluted somehow. Examples are solutions, where the drug is in solution at a given concentration, or a tablet, where for instance 100 mg of drug are present in a tablet weighing 300 mg.

The simplest of such cases of a diluted drug substance would be a powder, where the marketed product is a mixture of drug and other non-active substances, so-called *excipients*. In most such cases the drug is unstable in solution and a powder is supplied to the pharmacist for reconstitution. The pharmacist reconstitutes the powder with the prescribed amount of water, and gives it to the patient, cautioning that the material should be used up in the time period stated on the prescription.

There are cases where powders are sold in bottles[1] with a scoop and where the patient is then expected to take out one scoopful of powder, adding it to liquid and then ingesting the fluid product. One such case is Ques-

[1]They are also sold in pouches. Here the apparent density need not be controlled rigorously, as long as the correct amount of powder is present in each pouch, and the drug content of the powder blend is within acceptable limits.

tran (Mead-Johnson Div. of Bristol-Squibb). The active ingredient in Questran is cholestyramine, and the dose level is quite high (4 gm of cholestyramine resin). Such a large dose cannot be administered as a tablet or a capsule, and hence is dispensed as a powder, with the following precaution (PDR 35, p. 1149):

> The recommended adult dose is . . . one scoopful (containing 4 gm of cholestyramine resin in 9 grams of Questran) three or four times daily. . . . Questran should not be taken in its dry form. Always mix Questran powder with water or other fluids before ingesting. . . .

The pharmaceutical problem here is, that one scoopful must contain 4 gm of active, hence other ingredients must be added. Five grams are added to make the entire dose 9 grams, so that the product is a mixture.[2]

The physical adjustment that must be made is that the 9 grams must just fill the dispenser, which has a volume of 12 mL (cm^3). If the weight is divided by the volume, then a figure of 0.75 g/cm^3 results. This has the dimension of a density, but in actuality is not a true density, but an apparent density or bulk density. Some definitions are therefore in order.

True density is the mass (g) of a solid slab of a volume of 1 cm^3 (1 mL). It is determined experimentally by pycnometry, usually helium pycnometry. By this method a certain mass, M grams, of solid is introduced into a helium-filled vessel, and the amount of helium (V cm^3) it displaces is measured manometrically. The true density, ϱ, is then

$$\varrho = M/V \text{ g/cm}^3 \tag{2.3}$$

Since it is difficult to obtain a slab of solid of exactly 1 cm^3 volume, the density is usually obtained by pycnometry. This is illustrated by example below for a drug that is water-insoluble.

Example 2.1

Water is brought up to mark in a 25 cm^3 pycnometer (volumetric flask, with a spout as a stopper. Excess liquid is wiped off, and the contents are exactly 25 cm^3). The weight is 25.00 g. Now some of the water is removed and an accurately weighed sample of 1.20 gram of solid is added. The pycnometer is brought to volume with water weighed accurately and the weight found to be 25.4 g. Calculate the density of the solid.

---

[2]This could be adjusted chemically as well, in which case the product is not a mixture. It is assumed here, for the sake of example, that the product is a mixture of active and blank.

Answer 2.1

The following considerations are made.

The volume of water (after the addition of the solid) is 25 cm³ minus the volume of the solid, i.e.

$$25.0 - (1.2/\varrho) \tag{2.4}$$

This (since the density of water is 1.00, as determined in the first experiment) plus the weight of the solid equals the new weight, so that

$$25.4 = 1.2 + 25.0 - (1.2/\varrho) \tag{2.5}$$

from which it is seen that the true density is

$$26.2 - 25.4 = 0.8 = 1.2/\varrho \quad \text{or} \quad \varrho = 1.5 \text{ g/cm}^3 \tag{2.6}$$

Denoting by V the volume of the pycnometer, by ϱ_1 the density of the liquid and by ϱ_2 the density of the solid, the following equality exists, by a reasoning parallel to that above: The density of the liquid, ϱ_1, is found by filling it with the liquid and weighing it. If the weight of the pycnometer, containing M g of solid and q.s.'ed with liquid is W g, then there is $(W - M)$ g of liquid in the pycnometer, i.e., the volume of the liquid is:

$$V_1 = (W - M)/\varrho_1 \tag{2.7}$$

The volume of the solid is:

$$V_2 = M/\varrho_2 \tag{2.8}$$

The total volume is the sum of these two, i.e.

$$V = V_1 + V_2 = \{(W - M)/\varrho_1\} + \{M/\varrho_2\} \tag{2.9}$$

where only ϱ_2 is unknown.

If the volume of a scoop is V' (cm³), and the mass of material it contains is M' (g), then the apparent density [14] is given by:

$$\varrho' = M'/V' \text{ g/cm} \tag{2.10}$$

A sample of material that doesn't "fill" up the space, such as a scoop, is often referred to as a bed, and the fraction of the bed that is not solid (the void fraction), is called the *porosity*, usually denoted by the symbol ϵ. Since porosity in this definition is a fraction, it is dimensionless, and the number will be between 0 and 1.

It can be shown that the porosity is given by:

$$\epsilon = 1 - (\varrho'/\varrho) \tag{2.11}$$

Example 2.2

A powder consists of two components. Forty percent is one solid with a true density of 1.0 and 60% is a solid with a density of 1.5. A sample is poured into a 100 cm graduated cylinder, and the contents weigh 85 g. What is

(1) The average true density of the powder?
(2) The apparent density of the powder bed?
(3) The porosity of the powder bed?

Answer 2.2

(1) $(0.4 \times 1.0) + (0.6 \times 1.5) = 0.4 + 0.9 = 1.3$ gm/cm³
(2) $85/100 = 0.85$ gm/cm³
(3) $\epsilon = 1 - (0.85/1.3) = 0.35$

Aside from assuring that the mass of drug mixture in the scoop is correct, the powder mixture must be uniform, i.e., the drug content in each scoop should, ideally, be identical. This is utopian, and a certain range of contents is always unavoidable.

The following deals with the uniformity that one can expect to obtain in mixtures of two (or more) ingredients, and how such blending is accomplished. The USP uniformity test will be covered later.

2.3 NON-COHESIVE BLENDING (MIXING)

In the handling of powders, there are two types: cohesive powders and non-cohesive powders. We shall treat the latter first.

Mixing of non-cohesive powders takes place in different types of mixing equipment. The following is a list of the most common mixers used for non-cohesive powders:

(1) Barrel rollers
(2) Double helix trough-blender (ribbon blender)

(3) V-blenders

(4) Planetary mixers

These are illustrated in Figure 2.3.

All drug products have mixing steps as part of their manufacturing procedures. The FDA requires that a company validate the equipment and procedures used. The word "validation" denotes the experiment that proves that the equipment does what the company claims it does.

If a mixer is validated, it is necessary to somehow gauge how well the powder is blended. If, as in the Questran example above, the mixture is binary, and there is 4/9 of the drug and 5/9 of the excipient, then one may, of course, mix the two in the mixer in question, and assay the powder at different spots in the mixer from time to time. The better the mix is, the closer will be the results of the assays from the various parts of the mixer.

The composition, in blending validation, is usually expressed in fractions, x and $(1 - x)$, rather than in percentages. In the Questran example,

$$\text{the drug concentration is } x = 4/9 = 0.44 \text{ (or } 44\%) \qquad (2.12)$$

$$\text{the excipient concentration is } 0.56 \text{ (or } 56\%) \qquad (2.13)$$

It is conventional (and logical) to gauge the "perfection" of the mix by the standard deviation between the samples. If the samples are of the size of the

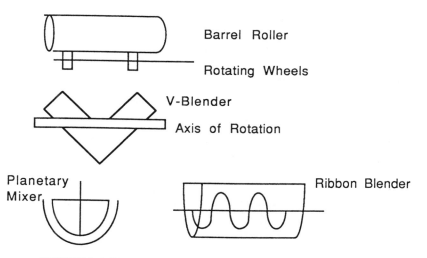

FIGURE 2.3. *Various types of mixers used for non-cohesive blending.*

dose (e.g., if they were 9 g samples in the case of Questran), and if ten samples are taken, then one may gauge the blending process by plotting the relative standard deviation (*RSD*) versus time in the mixer.

A set of results as shown in Table 2.1 might result. The variance of a set of numbers is defined as follows. If the numbers are denoted x_i, and if there are N of them, then the average is:

$$x_{avg} = \Sigma x_i / N \qquad (2.14)$$

e.g., for the 6-minute point in Table 2.1 (as shown in Table 2.2),

$$x_{avg} = (35 + 48 + 40 + 53)/4 = 176/4 = 44 \qquad (2.15)$$

(Note that, in a blending experiment, the average of the four need not be forty-four exactly, since there is also an uncertainty associated with the average.)

The variance of the set (s^2) is defined as

$$s^2 = \Sigma(x_i - x_{avg})^2/(N - 1) \qquad (2.16)$$

where N is the number of data points. The number $N - 1$ is denoted the degrees of freedom.

The standard deviation (s, or sd) is then the square root of this number, i.e.:

$$s = sd = [\Sigma(x_i - x_{avg})^2/(N - 1)]^{1/2} \qquad (2.17)$$

Example 2.3

Find the standard deviation for the set of assays after 6 minutes.

Answer 2.3

Table 2.2 shows the deviations. The variance is, therefore, $194/3 = 64.7$ and the standard deviation is $\sqrt{64.7} = 8$.

TABLE 2.1 Example of Blending Validation.

Time[a]	0	3	6	9
Assays[b]	0,100,0,100	19,59,38,65	35,48,40,53	46,37.8,42,44

[a]In minutes.
[b]In percent of active on a weight basis.

TABLE 2.2 Six-Minute Data from Table 2.1.

x_i	$(x_{avg} - x_i)$	$(x_{avg} - x_i)^2$
35	−9	81
48	+4	16
40	−4	16
53	+9	81
Sum 176	0	194

It is usual to use not the standard deviation, but the *relative standard deviation*. This latter is defined as:

$$RSD = 100 \times sd/x_{avg} \qquad (2.18)$$

i.e., in the above case, for 6 minutes, the relative standard deviation would be $100 \times 8/44 = 18.27\%$.

If the relative standard deviations for all the time points are calculated, then the situations shown in Table 2.3 and Figure 2.4 result.

It can be shown that the logarithms of the *RSD* values are linear in time. If the number of particles in the sample is large, then the blending equation becomes:

$$\ln [RSD] = -kt + \ln [RSD_o] \qquad (2.19)$$

This is shown in Table 2.4 and Figure 2.5. It will be seen in the next chapter, under content uniformity of capsules, that for a sample of ten units, the largest standard deviation permissible is 6%. This means that if the blending validation is carried out with ten samples (rather than four as in Table 2.1) and the sample size is exactly the weight (mass) of the dosage unit, then the blending should be carried out to the point where the *RSD* is no more than 6%.

It can be shown that the theoretical *initial RSD* is given by:

$$RSD_o = 100 [(1 - x)/x]^{1/2} \qquad (2.20)$$

For a powder that is later encapsulated, it is necessary that the relative

TABLE 2.3 Example of RSD Values from Table 2.1.

Time	0	3	6	9
RSD (%)	115	46.4	18.3	8.3

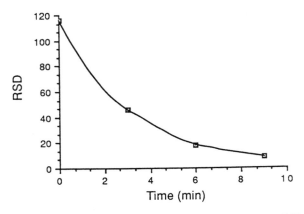

FIGURE 2.4. *RSD as a function of blending time. Data from Table 2.1.*

standard deviation be less than 6% when ten samples are taken, and the sample size must equal that of the dosage form weight.

It can also be shown that blending cannot be carried out to a *RSD* of less than:

$$RSD_\infty = 100 \left[(1 - x)/\{Nx\} \right] \tag{2.21}$$

where *N* is the number of particles in the dosage form. Since *N* is usually very large, this number is most often close to zero.

2.4 PREBLENDING

The blending rate constant, k, in Equation (2.19) is a function of the fraction of drug in the mixture. When there is less than 50% of drug (i.e., $x < 0.5$), then the relation is given by:

$$k' = 2k_{50}x \tag{2.22}$$

where k_{50} is the blending rate constant (the slope of the line) when the drug content is 50%.

TABLE 2.4 Blending Data Presented Semi-Logarithmically.

Time	0	3	6	9
ln [RSD]	4.74	3.83	2.90	2.11

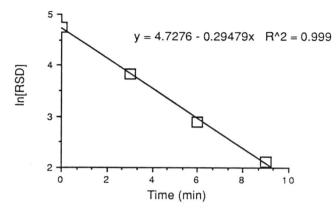

FIGURE 2.5. *ln [RSD] as a function of time. Data from Table 2.4.*

Direct blending can be done as long as there is more than 10% active in the blend. With less than 10% (but more than 1%), preblending is resorted to. Preblending means that the drug is blended with a portion of the excipient(s) and this preblend is then mixed with the remainder of the excipient(s). This is best illustrated by example.

Example 2.4

Five kg of drug substance is to be blended with 95 kg of excipient to give 100 kg of mixture containing 5% of drug. Suggest a preblending scheme.

Answer 2.4

For instance, the 5 kg of drug could be mixed with 20 kg of one of the excipients to form 25 kg of preblend. The 25 kg of preblend would then be mixed with the remaining 75 kg of excipients to form the 100 kg of final blend.

It can be shown [15] that the best total amount of preblend is given by $\sqrt{x}$, so that in the above example, since $x = 0.05$, the best total amount of preblend would be $\sqrt{0.05} = 0.223$, i.e., 22.3%, so that 5 kg of drug would be mixed with 17.3 kg of excipient to form 22.3 kg of preblend, and this would then be final-blended with the remaining 77.7 kg of excipients.

This optimum ratio gives the smallest blending time to achieve a given standard deviation, but often preblend sizes are a function of available equipment. They are often carried out in barrel rollers.

When the amounts of drug are less than 1% (or 0.1% a bit depending on the drug substance), it becomes uncomfortable to even preblend. Preblend-ing could then be done geometrically, i.e., 1 part drug to 1 part excipient, then 1 part first preblend with 1 part excipient, then 1 part second preblend with 1 part excipient, and so on until all has been blended. This is cumber-some, although it is often done on a laboratory scale.

On larger scale, such high-potency drugs are most often dissolved in a solvent and added to the excipients. In this manner the liquid distributes evenly over the excipient particles, and there is theoretically an ideal con-tent uniformity ($SD = 0$). This is not quite true, as shall be mentioned later, but it comes close to the truth. This is the manner in which ethinyles-tradiol is added in many contraceptive products.

2.5 SEGREGATION

Non-cohesive particles will segregate when there is a large difference be-tween the particle sizes. In the simplest case there are two ingredients, A and B, each with a different particle diameter, d_A and d_B (see Figure 2.6).

- If $d_A = d_B$, then blending is fast [16], and segregation does not take place.
- If $d_A > d_B$, but B does not fit into the interstices in A, then blend-ing is virtually impossible [16]. If blending is accomplished by stacking, then segregation is rapid [17].
- If $d_A > d_B$, but B can fit into the interstices in A, then blending is fast, and segregation is fast [16].

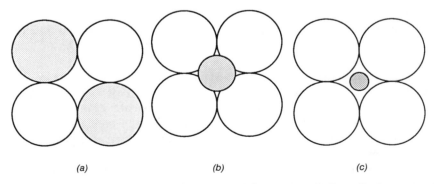

FIGURE 2.6. Blending situations [16]: (a) A and B same size; (b) B smaller but cannot percolate; (c) B smaller but can percolate.

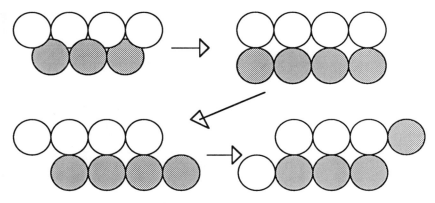

FIGURE 2.7. *Blending of powders. At first the particles are in a close arrangement. There is a bed expansion as a first step, into a loose configuration, then the layers move relative to one another, and finally there is vertical movement, initiating the actual blending.*

2.6 COHESION AND FRICTION

In the above it is assumed that C is minimal. The blending then consists of simply making sure that the particles rearrange from a close packing (Figure 2.7) to a loose packing so that they can move with respect to one another [18].

The blending rate is a function of the frictional force between the particles, and of the cohesive stresses involved. To appreciate the concept of friction, consider a body placed on a plane, such as shown in Figure 2.8. The relation between the tangential force, τ, and the normal force, σ, is:

$$\tau = \mu\sigma \qquad (2.23)$$

where μ is called the frictional coefficient.

When powders are cohesive, a force must be applied to "pry them apart," and this force must equal or supersede the cohesional force. It has been mentioned that the angle of repose is an indication of the cohesive forces in a powder. The larger the angle the larger the cohesive force.

If powder is allowed to flow out upon a plane surface (Figure 2.9), then the side of the cone forms an angle of α, the repose angle, with the plane.

It is noted that a particle at A on the surface of the cone is subjected to two forces: the gravitational force, mg, depicted by arrow AD, and the cohesional force, c, denoted by AC. If AD is divided up by a force parallelogram, then the component in the normal direction is AB. Since angle BEA

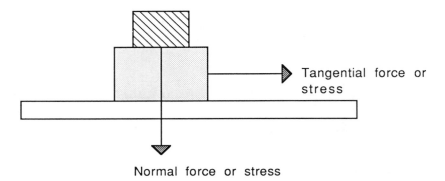

Tangential force or
stress

Normal force or stress

FIGURE 2.8. Schematic of friction. The tangential force is τ and the normal force (stress) is σ.

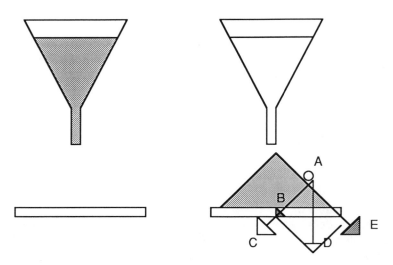

FIGURE 2.9. Powder flowing through a funnel, and forming a heap on the plane. The force parallelogram is shown in the cone.

is α, it follows that the magnitude of AB is mg cos $[\alpha]$. The normal force is hence

$$\sigma = c + \text{mg cos } [\alpha] \qquad (2.24)$$

The tangential force is by a similar argument AE, which equals

$$\tau = \text{mg sin } [\alpha] \qquad (2.25)$$

Since the situation is such that the particle is just about to move, Equation (2.23) holds, i.e.

$$\text{mg sin } [\alpha] = \mu(c + \text{mg cos } [\alpha]) \qquad (2.26)$$

Equation (2.26) shows that the larger c is, the larger α is (i.e., the more cohesive the powder is, the larger the repose angle). It is not possible, however, to find both c and μ quantitatively, because Equation (2.26) is one equation with two unknowns. Actual determination of these quantities will be discussed later.

2.7 COHESIVE BLENDING. ORDERED MIXING

If the two powders that are to be blended are cohesive, then the cohesive force must be overcome during the mixing. In the mixers listed previously (as-is), the forces created by the mixing will usually not suffice to overcome the cohesive force, so that the cohesive powder (which is lumpy), will fall apart into smaller lumps, but not into the prime particles.

This is usually overcome by placing a rotor (impeller) in the mixer (high intensity blenders, e.g., Collette or Lödige mixers or running a V-blender with intensifier bars). In this case the mixer simply serves to pass the powder over the rotor, where the force intensity is high. This breaks apart the lumps, and excipient particles will lodge themselves in between the drug particles and keep them separated.

If the drug particles are sufficiently smaller than the excipient particles, then so-called *ordered mixing* can result. Here the cohesive force (due to the small size of the drug particle) keeps the small particles almost glued to the large particles (Figure 2.10). Segregation does not occur in such situations [19].

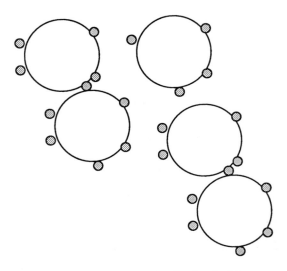

FIGURE 2.10. *Schematic of ordered mixing.*

2.8 REFERENCES

1. Carstensen, J. T. and P.-C. Chan. 1976. *Powder Tech.*, 15:129.
2. Pilpel, N. 1964. *J. Pharm. Pharmacol.*, 16:705.
3. Nelson, E. 1955. *J. Am. Pharm. Assoc.*, *Sci., Ed.*, 44:435.
4. Neuman, B. 1967. *Adv. Pharm. Sci.*, 2:181.
5. Carstensen, J. T. and P.-C. Chan. 1976. *J. Pharm. Sci.*, 65:1235.
6. Pilpel, N. 1973. *Adv. Pharm. Sci.*, 3:174.
7. Bradley, R. S. 1936. *Trans. Faraday Soc.*, 32:1088.
8. Hamaker, H. C. 1937. *Physica*, 4:1058.
9. Hiestand, E. 1966. *J. Pharm. Sci.*, 55:1235.
10. Jordan, D. W. 1954. *J. Appl. Phys.*, 5:S194.
11. Carr, R. L. 1965. *Chem. Eng.*, 72(2):163.
12. Kaneniwa, N., A. Ikekawa and H. Aoki. 1967. *Chem. Pharm. Bull.*, 15:1441.
13. Nogami, H. J., M. Sugiwara and S. Kimura. 1965. *Yakuzaigaku*, 25:260.
14. Holman, L. E. and H. Leuenberger. 1990. *Powder Tech.*, 60:249.
15. Carstensen, J. T. and C. T. Rhodes. 1984. *Drug Dev. Ind., Pharm.*, 10:1017.
16. Carstensen, J. T. and M. R. Patel. 1977. *Powder Technology*, 17:273.
17. Rippie, E. G., J. L. Olsen and M. D. Faiman. 1964. *J. Pharm. Sci.*, 53:1360.
18. Malhotre, K., A. S. Mujumdar, H. Imakoma and M. Okazak. 1988. *Powder Tech.*, 55:107.
19. Hersey, J. A. 1975. *Powder Technology*, 1:94.

2.9 PROBLEMS (CHAPTER 2)*

(1) Tetracycline is blended with citric acid to be encapsulated at a fill weight of 400 mg. The capsules are to contain 250 mg of tetracycline. Neither of the two substances are cohesive. They are monodisperse and both have the same particle size.

   The powders are mixed in a blender. Four-hundred mg samples are taken from ten spots at two time points (5 and 10 minutes blending). The samples are assayed chemically and the results (expressed as mg of tetracycline per 400 mg) are listed below:

5 min	224	200	316	156	356	216	332	172	308	220
10 min	240	220	256	248	308	252	248	216	252	260

   (a) List the standard deviation (in mg/400 mg) and the relative standard deviation at the two time points.
   (b) What is the blending rate constant? Give units.
   (c) Assuming that the finished capsules would have the same uniformity as the mixture, how long would the powder have to be mixed in the blender to pass a USP content uniformity test at the first try (i.e., testing only ten units and not going to the additional twenty unit assay)?
   (d) If the mixture were blended to a relative standard deviation of 7.8%, would it pass the USP content uniformity test on resampling (i.e., assaying twenty more capsules)?

*Answers on page 235.

CHAPTER 3

Hard Shell Capsules and Apparent Densities

As mentioned in Chapter 2, the next least complicated of solid dosage forms (in regards to simplicity of formation) is the hard shell capsule. The empty hard shells are purchased from manufacturers (Capsugel, Elanco) and may be filled by hand if need be. Newer machines (Häffliger-Karg, Zannazi) in a way imitate the hand-filling of capsules. The less modern three-ring (Colton) capsule machine does not.

3.1 HARD SHELL CAPSULE MACHINES

This latter is the simplest (and the oldest) of the machines and is a two-ring filling principle. The powder is placed in a movable hopper (Figure 3.1). The capsules themselves are in a stationary hopper (not shown in Figure 3.1). When the machine is turned on, capsules will fall through a chute, align themselves, and drop into a split ring. By means of vacuum the bodies of the capsules are sucked into the lower ring, and the caps stay in the top ring. The rings are then separated and the lower part placed on a turntable. As the table turns, the powder flows from the hopper into the body of the capsules. When all the capsules in the ring (B) are filled, the hopper is moved back, the turntable (if need be) is stopped and the two rings brought together again. By means of a pegboard (D) (Figure 3.2), the capsules are then (a) pushed together while the plate A is placed behind the B and C rings (i.e., the body is re-entered into the cap) and (b) the plate A is removed, and D is pushed all the way, so that the pegs eject the now-closed capsules.

The method is fairly slow, and more rapid methods are used in production nowadays. However the three-ring machine is quite adequate and practical for product development of initial clinical batches, which often use quite small amounts of raw material.

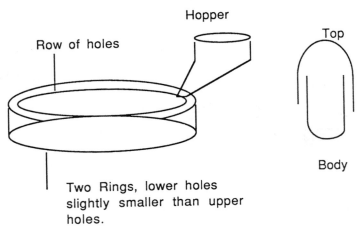

FIGURE 3.1. *Two-ring hard shell machine, showing the powder hopper and the filling ring.*

The hopper is equipped with an auger, and this pushes the powder (gently) into the shell. The faster the machine goes, the less time the auger has to "push" and the less time the powders have to flow and, hence, the lower the fill weight. This is, as shall be seen, only true up to a certain point. The effect of flow, apparent density, and die volume is more conveniently covered under tablets.

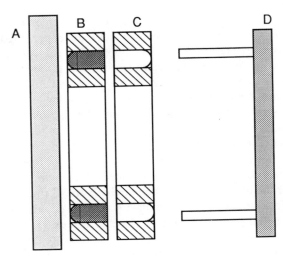

FIGURE 3.2. *Pegboard capsule joining and ejection.*

Dosator machines, as the name implies, rely on a dosator. This is a cylinder with a movable base. The powder is stomped into the cavity by the downwards stroke of the dosator (see Figure 3.3). (Application of vacuum is also possible on certain machines.) The amount of material filled into this cavity (the fill weight) is a function of the particle size distribution and compressibility of the powder. Since a plug must be formed (otherwise the powder would flow back out when the dosator is removed from the powder bed) the powder must have some cohesion. Hence, from a formulation point of view it differs from the considerations that must be given to capsules made on a two-ring machine. The HK and Zannasi machines have a special arrangement for separating the two capsule shells, the dosator delivers the plug to the body of the capsule, and the top is then applied.

3.2 FACTORS OTHER THAN FLOW AFFECTING THE FILL

The most important factor affecting the fill is the apparent density of the powder at the degree of compression afforded either by the auger in the two-ring machine or the dosator in the other machines.

If a powder is filled into a volume and gently compressed (below its elastic limit), then it will reduce in volume, i.e., the apparent density will increase. In the capsule this has the effect of "pushing" on the side of the capsule wall of the body of the capsule, so that when the capsule is closed in the pegboard operation, it will be under tension, i.e., tight. Obviously this pressure cannot

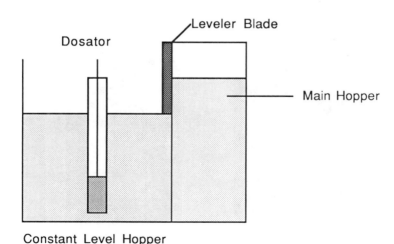

FIGURE 3.3. Dosator principle.

be too great, since then the powder would "pop out" of the body of the capsule when it passed by the hopper. On storage, the top could be pushed off of the body by the elastic expansion. In a given pressure range, however, the capsule has the desired degree of tightness.

The actual fill achievable is the compacted apparent density, r^*, times the volume V of the body of the hard shell. The precision of the fill is partly a function of the flow rate and of the fineness of the powder. If the powder is too coarse (Figure 3.4), then the fill will be erratic, when it is too fine the flow will be poor, so that a compromise is usually reached (i.e., some intermittent particle size that gives sufficiently accurate fill weights and does not impair flow too much).

A formula for a hard shell capsule product may be as simple as the following three ingredients:

(1) Drug Substance
(2) Filler (e.g., lactose hydrate)
(3) Lubricant (e.g., magnesium stearate) 0.5–1%

The lubricant is added to facilitate the hopper movement back and forth over the fill ring. The amount used is rarely over 1%, since large amounts of lubricant interfere with dissolution.

In a simplified way of looking at formulation, the first thing to be established is what the fill weight should be. If 250 mg of drug is to be filled into the capsule, but if this only fills up the capsule say 2/3 of the way, then the remainder must be taken up with filler.

Capsule shells come in different sizes (Table 3.1), and the smallest capsule volume for say, a 250 mg (0.25 g) dose of a drug with an apparent density of

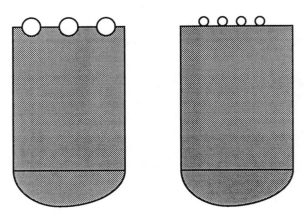

FIGURE 3.4. *Coarse and fine powder fill.*

TABLE 3.1 Capsule Sizes.

Capsule Size	0	1	2	3	4	5
Volume (mL)	0.68	0.50	0.37	0.30	0.21	0.13

0.8 g/cm³ would be 0.25/0.8 = 0.31 cm³. Hence, from Table 3.1, a #2 capsule can be used, a #4 capsule cannot be used, and a #3 capsule would be cutting it close. Just because the particular lot of drug in hand has an apparent density of 0.8 does not mean that the next batch will be that dense. One may, in bulk powders, assume a variation in bulk density of 5% or more, even for manufacturing processes that are well in control.

Assuming that for a variety of reasons (one being marketing) it has been decided in the above case to proceed with a #1 capsule, then a very oversimplified mode of approaching the problem of anticipated fill weight would be as follows: the drug has an apparent density of 0.8 g/cm³, and, as a general rule, many excipients (e.g., lactose in certain particle size ranges) have an apparent density about that, as well. If one then further assumes that a mixture of excipient and drug has an apparent density of 0.8 g/cm³, then knowing the volume of the capsule, one may calculate the fill weight. In this case, a #1 capsule has a volume of 0.5 cm³ and the powder an apparent density of 0.8 g/cm³, so that the amount to be filled under these circumstances would be 0.8 × 0.5 = 0.4 g, or 400 mg. Since 250 mg are drug, 150 mg would be the amount of excipient to use. If one assumes 1/2% magnesium stearate to be added (2 mg), then 150 − 2 = 148 mg would be lactose, giving the *provisional* composition of the capsule fill.

From a manufacturing point of view, two batches are never going to have the same apparent density and compressibility, so that under the same conditions, the fill weight would be different in the two batches. The two-ring capsule machine, however, can be run at different speeds. A higher speed gives less of a chance for powder to flow into the capsule, and the action of the auger is in play for less time since the contact time between the capsule and the hopper is shorter. Hence the machine speed can (within limits) be used to achieve the correct fill weight.

Suppose, in the above case, the actual fill weight had been 420 mg—then the machine could be run a bit faster, and the speed found at which 400 mg would be the fill weight. Conversely if the fill weight had been 380 mg, then the machine could be run more slowly. Such variation can however not exceed 10–15%, and if for example the actual fill weight had been found to be 500 mg, then reformulation would be necessary. The first attempt would be to use 2.5 mg of magnesium stearate and 250 − 2.5 = 247.5 mg of lactose. However, things are not quite that simple, as shall be seen shortly. For instance, apparent densities are not additive. What is most often done is a trial and error approach, and a statement that the amount of filler may be varied if necessary (and giving the limits of such a variation). Wet granulation will be covered later, and at times (particularly in Europe) the powder is "standardized" by wet granulating it, so that (with this process always producing fairly much the same particle size distribution) the fill weight will be set. The granulation also helps the flow.

With capsules based on the dosator principle, the fill weight can be adjusted directly with the dosator. Here the fill weight is a function of both the position of the plunger in the dosator and the level of the powder bed in the constant level portion of the machine. Flow is important here because good flow will ascertain a smooth level in the leveling compartment, whereas erratic and poor flow will not, and the latter condition will give rise to fill weight variation. (The fill weight is a function of the level of powder in the leveling compartment.)

In recent years dosage forms have been attempted where there is a liquid fill into the capsule [1,2] (e.g., PEG bases). These go under the name of "liquid-filled caplets" in the over-the-counter market in the U.S.

Recent reviews of hard capsule technology have appeared in the literature [3,4].

3.3 APPARENT DENSITY AND PARTICLE SIZES

For simplicity it shall be assumed that the capsule powder consists of a coarse component, C, and a fine component, F. If a sample of powder of the coarse component is placed in a 100 mL graduate, then a situation such as shown in Figure 3.5 results. If the fine powder can percolate then addition of it will simply fill up the void space, and the mass (M) will increase without the volume $(V = 100$ mL$)$ increasing, so that the apparent density becomes:

$$r' = (M_A + M_B)/V \tag{3.1}$$

The apparent density will reach its maximum when the entire void space in the coarse powder is filled up with fine powder, and if more fine powder is added, the powder will consist of coarse powder particles suspended evenly in a bed of fine powder [5–7].

If the apparent density is plotted as a function of fraction of fines, then a plot as shown in Figure 3.6 will result. It can be shown that if the reciprocals of the apparent densities (the apparent volumes) are plotted, then a graph ensues (Figure 3.7) which consists of two line segments that intersect at the maximum density composition. It is seen in Figure 3.7 that the intersection of

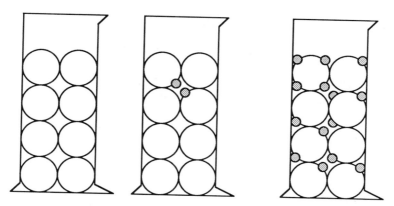

FIGURE 3.5. *Apparent density and powder composition.*

the "above max line" with the y-axis at a value that is the reciprocal of the true density of the coarse powder. The "below max line" cuts the x-axis at the point of 100%.

The points B and C, of course, represent the reciprocal of the apparent densities of the coarse and the fine powder.

Hard shell capsules come in several sizes, given in Table 3.1. Sometimes the shape of the capsule is of importance. Elanco and Pharmagel capsules have slightly different radii of curvature in the bottom of the body of the capsule. It is, at times, sufficiently important that they are not interchangeable for certain formulations (and may not fit in, e.g., blisters of the same die cut).

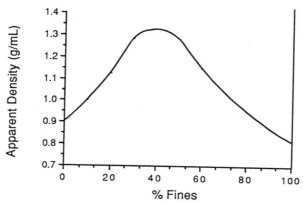

FIGURE 3.6. *Apparent density of a binary, bidisperse mixture, as a function of fraction of fines.*

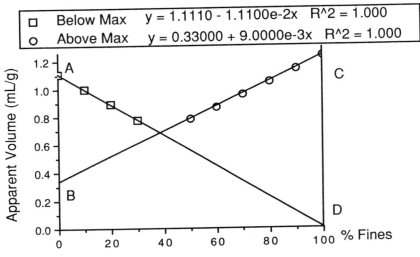

FIGURE 3.7. *Apparent volumes as a function of fines content.*

Capsules are most frequently printed for identification (company and strength), and can have different colors (e.g., top one color, body another). Capsules can be snap-locks, i.e., due to a slight groove, once they are closed they cannot be opened (easily) again. They can also be banded. These steps serve both as anti-tampering and identification.

Some capsules are bullet-shaped, i.e., there is a taper in the lower end of the body of the capsule.

3.4 FACTORS AFFECTING MACHINE OPERATION

Gelatin is somewhat hygroscopic, and operations must be carried out at relative humidities lower than 40% RH, otherwise the capsule parts will stick together and affect the body/cap separation operations.

The gelatin has the correct "consistency" if it contains 11–17% moisture. Above that it becomes soft and deforms, and below that it becomes brittle. There are several types of gelatin, e.g., the sources vary (pork or calf) as does the processing, being either alkaline or acid. The gelatins hence have different isoelectric points so that the 11/17% figures should be interpreted with some caution.

The hygroscopicity of gelatin can also be a factor in the storage performance, since if a powder is more hygroscopic than the gelatin, then it can pull moisture out of the capsule shell, which then becomes brittle. This will be discussed further in Chapter 12.

3.5 SOFT SHELL CAPSULES

In soft shell capsules (Figure 3.8) two sheets of gelatin are formed into pockets, and (in the case of liquid-filled soft shell capsules) a liquid is dosed into the cavity just prior to sealing. The gelatin films are a solution of water, gelatin, and glycerin. After the (wet) capsule has been formed, it is dried to a given moisture content. This cannot be too low, since then the capsule would be brittle, or too high, since then it would distort in storage. The glycerin content is also critical, since too small a content would contribute to brittleness, and too large a content to distortability.

The fill is usually a triglyceride (oil) or polyethylene glycol (PEG, Carbowax). Oils are completely immiscible with the shell, but PEG presents a problem in that the glycerin is soluble in it, and to compensate for this, an equilibrium amount of glycerin is usually added to the fill to prevent glycerin from leaving the shell.

R. P. Scherer essentially has a monopoly on this type of dosage form in the United States. Some solids are stabilized in oil solution, others in solutions of polyethylene glycol (e.g., several prostaglandins), so that soft shell capsules are a good dosage form for such products. Furthermore, dyes can provide light screening in the correct wavelength range and protect light-sensitive entities.

Titanium dioxide is used as the most common opacifier. (Iron oxides are also used.) The titanium dioxide is opaque and if considered completely non-transparent (see Figure 3.9) will lengthen the pathway of light passing through the capsule, so that more light will be absorbed, hence the product will be better protected from light.

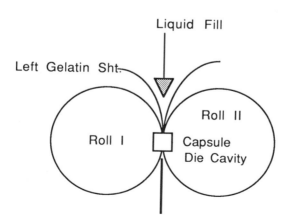

FIGURE 3.8. Soft liquid fill capsules.

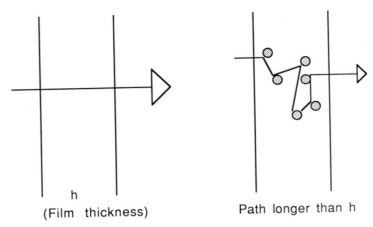

(Film thickness)   Path longer than h

FIGURE 3.9. *Light protection afforded by increased path length in an opaque hard shell capsule.*

When the capsule is formed, the gelatin films are wet (and they are dried subsequently). There is always a migration, to some degree, of water or gelatin/glycerin soluble excipients or drugs into the shell, and this migration is a function of the type of gelatin used [8].

3.6 DISSOLUTION OF CAPSULES

3.6.1 Disintegration and Dissolution of Capsules and Tablets

Capsules when tested by USP Method #2 (Paddle) are usually weighted down with a metal coil, so they will sink. Upon storage, the powder, if it is sufficiently hygroscopic, may pull out moisture from the capsule shell, and "granulate," i.e., agglomerate. This may slow down dissolution (decrease, for instance, the amount dissolved after 30 minutes). Most quality control specifications are "one-point" tests, e.g., the USP often specifies that 75% must dissolve after 30 minutes. If, for instance, in the dissolution of a 0.5 gram tablet the length of time for 75% (0.375 grams) to dissolve has increased from 2 to 6 minutes in 1 year's storage, it can be shown (not shown here) that after 2 years the length of time required to dissolve 75% of the drug may increase to about 30 minutes.

Gelatin capsules have a water content of 12–14%. If the equilibrium water vapor pressure of the capsule powder is considerably lower than that of the gelatin, then so much of the water can be drawn out of the shell that (1) the shell becomes brittle, and (2) the moisture added to the powder granulates it completely so that it becomes a hard plug. In such a case, the dissolution of the drug will be a square root law (treated in Chapter 15).

3.7 REFERENCES

1. Bowtle, W. J., N. J. Barker and J. Woodham. 1988. *Pharm. Techn.*, 12:862.
2. Cole, E. T. 1989. *Pharm. Techn.*, 13:124.
3. Ridgway, K. 1987. *Hard Capsules, Development and Technology.* London, UK: The Pharmaceutical Press.
4. Augsberger, L. L. 1988. *J. Pharm. Sci.*, 8:734.
5. Carstensen, J. T., F. Puisieux, A. Mehta and M. A. Zoglio. 1978. *Powder Tech.*, 20:2492.
6. Carstensen, J. T. 1977. *Pharmaceutics of Solids and Solid Dosage Forms.* New York, NY: Wiley, pp. 138–140.
7. Carstensen, J. T. 1980. *Solid Pharmaceutics: Mechanical Properties and Rate Phenomena.* New York, NY: Academic Press, p. 72.

3.8 PROBLEMS (CHAPTER 3)*

(1) Ibuprofen is insoluble in water. A volumetric flask with a graded neck is filled to the 25 mL mark with water. The contents weigh 25 grams. 1.592 grams of ibuprofen are added to the liquid, and the level of the liquid rises to 26.1 mL.

    (a) What is the true density of ibuprofen? (Use three significant figures, i.e., two digits after the decimal point.)

Ibuprofen powder is poured into a 50 mL graduate up to the 50 mL mark. The contents weigh 45.69 grams.

    (b) What is the apparent density of ibuprofen?

    (c) What is the porosity of the powder bed?

    (d) You want to fill 400 mg of ibuprofen into a capsule. Which capsule size is the smallest you can use? (Assume no compression during the encapsulation.)

    (e) After having selected your capsule size, you wish to add lactose as a diluent. Assume that both lactose and ibuprofen are spherical particles with a diameter of 100 μm. What is the amount of lactose you would add? (Lactose has true density of 1.45 g/cm³.)

    (f) If the powder is blended to completion, what would be the smallest relative standard deviation attainable with this mix?

*Answers on pages 236, 237.

(g) If you had used a capsule one size larger than the one you selected, what would your relative standard deviation have been?

(2) A drug product is marketed as a 15 and a 30 mg capsule. It is desired to perform a special clinical study of a capsule containing 60 mg of drug substance in a #4 capsule (volume 0.21 cm³). Assume you can do this with the simplest possible composition, using lactose and magnesium stearate, and assume that the apparent density of each of these ingredients is 0.8 g/cm³. The capsules are to be encapsulated on a two-ring machine. Assume drug, magnesium stearate, and lactose to be both free of lumps and fairly non-cohesive.

    (a) If you assume that a mixture of the powders has the same apparent density as the individual powders, what is the first composition of the capsule powder you would try? (Use 1/2% magnesium stearate.)

    (b) The size of the clinical order is 10,000 capsules. You decide to make enough powder for two rings to see if the formula works satisfactorily. There are 104 "holes" (capsules) per ring. What is the formula (the actual amount weighed out of each ingredient) for this amount of powder?

    (c) You run your trial and find the following weights of the contents of ten capsules:

178, 180, 185, 176, 171, 178, 181, 184, 175, and 172 mg

What is the average drug content per capsule? (Show short calculation.)

Would you run the machine faster to get the right weight, run the machine more slowly to get the right weight, or reformulate the powder?

    (d) If your trial run had given the following weights of the contents of ten capsules:

198, 200, 205, 196, 211, 198, 201, 204, 195, and 192 mg.

What would have been the average drug content per capsule? (Show short calculation.)

Would you run the machine faster to get the right weight, run the machine more slowly to get the right weight, or reformulate the powder?

    (e) If the answer is #3 in either case, suggest a formula (amounts per capsule) that might give the correct average drug content.

    (f) Suppose your first formula [step (a)] gave the correct fill weight and you now were to make the 10,000 capsules. Why shouldn't you preblend? (One-line answer.)

(g) You blend the mixture for 4 and 6 minutes in a planetary mixer and obtain the following assays for drug from ten different spots, the sample size being the same as the theoretical fill weight of your capsules:

4 min 70, 23, 97, 21, 99, 50, 45, 75, 33, 87
6 min 60, 43, 77, 36, 84, 60, 51, 69, 38, 82

(1) What is the blending rate constant?
(2) What is the relative standard deviation at time zero as calculated from the data?
(3) What should it be, theoretically?
(4) How long should you mix in order that the capsules would meet USP specifications?

(h) It was stated in the preamble to the problem that the lactose was non-cohesive. Yet, in the laboratory, it was quite evident that the lactose used was quite cohesive. If the sample used in this problem is indeed non-cohesive, what could be the reason? (One-line answer.)

CHAPTER 4

Milling (Comminution)

Early in product development, when only small amounts of drug are available, comminution may be carried out with a mortar and pestle. This step also accomplishes deagglomeration in the case of cohesive powders. For small batches mortar and pestle mixing/milling is quite suitable, but for larger batches it is not practical due to the length of time required.

4.1 BALL MILLING

The oldest means of grinding are millstones, but ball mills are probably very old as well. One of the tasks of milling is to reduce the particle size, without changing the characteristics of the powder in any other way. It will be seen in a later chapter that crystal structure and crystallinity are important attributes of a pharmaceutical powder (drug substances in particular), and at the onset it should be pointed out that ball milling in particular (and other types of milling in sensitive cases) can change the morphology of a solid, e.g., make a crystalline compound amorphous [1–4]. Strong grinding can give a solid an increase in the surface energy [5,6], and can distort the crystal lattice [7,8].

The milling equipment that is traditionally used in intermediate batch sizes (e.g., up to 100 g, in most instances) is a small ball mill.

A ball mill is shown in Figure 4.1. It is usually made out of porcelain, and the balls themselves can be either porcelain or stainless steel.

The number of balls, the rotational speed, and the amount of powder and the length of time of milling are factors that affect how well the powder is milled.

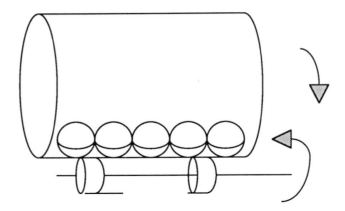

FIGURE 4.1. *Ball mill.*

When the rotational speed is small, then the balls cascade one over the other, thus causing the grinding action. At higher rotational speeds the balls "climb up" the walls of the mill and fall into the material from their apex, thus causing grinding by impact.

Increasing the speed in this region increases the efficiency of milling up to a point. It is clear, however, that the speed at which the balls start "centrifuging" onto the wall is the highest allowable speed.

This happens [9] at an angular velocity, u (in radians per second), given by:

$$u = [2g/D]^{1/2} \qquad (4.1)$$

where D is the diameter of the mill, and g is the gravitational acceleration.

The usual rotational speeds of ball mills are 50–80% of the critical speed, u. The optimum speed of a ball mill is

$$v = 78 - 40(\ln [D]) \qquad (4.2)$$

Smaller balls give a finer grinding, but require longer time to achieve the degree grinding of a given charge. The optimum diameter, δ, of a ball in a given mill is, k being a constant [1]

$$\delta = k[D]^{1/2} \qquad (4.3)$$

In a ball mill (usually porcelain), balls are placed with the powder in a cylinder, and this is then rotated by being placed on a set of rotating wheels.

The longer the time of milling, the faster (below the centrifugal speed) the rotational speed; and the larger the ratio of ball weight to powder weight, the higher the degree of comminution, i.e., the finer the powder will be.

The energy, E, expended in milling w grams of powder, is given by Kick's law [9–11] which states that:

$$E = C \cdot \ln [d'/d''] \qquad (4.4)$$

where C is a constant, d' is the diameter of the incoming powder, and d'' is the diameter of the milled powder. If this consists of two fractions, one of w_a of diameter d' (which is the part that essentially was not milled) and one, w_b g of diameter d_b cm (the milled fraction, $1 - f'$), then

$$d'' = (w_a d' + w_b d_b)/w \qquad (4.5)$$

where f' is the fraction not milled. Inserting Equation (4.4) into (4.5) and noting that the amount of energy input is proportional to time ($E = qt$, where q is a constant), gives:

$$E = qt = -C \cdot \ln \{(w_a/w) + (w_b d_b/wd')\} \qquad (4.6)$$

At short milling times this simplifies to:

$$\ln (w/w_a) = -(q/C)t \qquad (4.7)$$

so that the fraction not milled is an exponential decay in time [10,11].

4.2 HAMMER MILLS

Although ball milling on a large scale is possible, it is virtually never used in the pharmaceutical industry. Rather, hammer milling is used (Figure 4.2). Powder is bled into the mill house via the hopper, and the rotating hammers impact with the powder. When this is fine enough to pass the screen, it will exit. The powder exiting will have a maximum particle size of that of the screen. Description of particle sizes and distributions will be made in Chapter 14, but suffice it now to say that the average particle size of the milled powder will be smaller, the smaller the feed rate, the more rapid the milling speed (rpm's), and the finer the screen. The knife has a blunt edge on one side and a knife edge on the other. Milling with the blunt edge forward gives rise to a smaller average particle size. Finally, not all

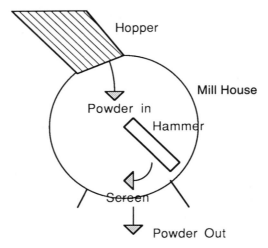

FIGURE 4.2. *Hammer mill.*

powders behave similarly, and milling conditions satisfactory for one drug product may not be satisfactory for another.

The efficiency of a hammer mill is not large, so a great deal of heat is built up during the operation. For heat-sensitive products, cooling coils can be placed in the mill house, or solid dry ice may be added to the powder mixture. These procedures have a tendency to cause moisture condensation from the atmosphere, and if cooling (indirect or direct) is employed, the relative humidity of the milling room should be kept as low as possible.

The usual minimum particle range is about 50 μm. Large, heavy-duty hammer mills, so-called micropulverizers, can bring the particle size further down (typically to 20 μm). If particle sizes less than 5 μm are desired, micronizers are used. These will be described shortly.

4.3 PARTICLE SIZES FROM HAMMER MILLING

If a powder contains only particles of one size, then it is denoted *monodisperse*, otherwise it is denoted *polydisperse*. If a powder sample, even if it were monodisperse, were milled, then it would be fortuitous if all the particles emerging from the mill would be of the same size. Hence, milled powders are, as a rule, polydisperse.

The particles are finer than the material before it was milled. Figure 4.3 shows the trajectory of a particle as it is leaving the mill, and it is obvious

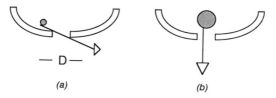

FIGURE 4.3. *Particle leaving the screen opening in a mill: (a) trajectory forms an angle with the screen; (b) not perpendicular.*

that the diameter after (d_{af}) is smaller than the hole in the screen (D). Hence it would be fallacious to estimate the actual particle size of the milled particle as being equal to the size of the opening in the screen. Furthermore, if the hammer speed is large, then the angle will be more shallow, and the effective opening will be smaller. This is one of the reasons that high hammer speed causes smaller particles. Having knives forward, rather than blunt edge, probably affects the actual speed of the particle, so that this is one of the reasons that blunt edge forward gives finer particles. The other main reason is, of course, the impact of hammer on the particle, which is higher at high speed and with blunt edge forward. Finally, high speed causes more turbulence in the chamber, and self-attrition of the particles (the particles breaking by collision with one another) also becomes more pronounced.

Figure 4.4 shows an example of the size of the emerging powder as a function of the opening in the screen [12]. In the case cited, the screens used were solid metal screens with large holes, and the powder milled fairly

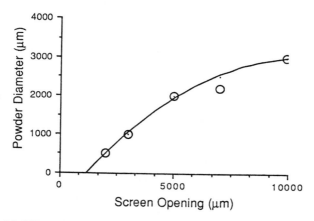

FIGURE 4.4. *Effect of screen opening size on the average particle size of the milled powder.*

coarse. To characterize the "mean diameter," the so-called weight mean diameter, d, can be obtained from sieve (screen) test.

4.4 ATTRITION MILLS

If particle sizes in the micron range are required, then the powder is usually micronized. Here particles are bled into a chamber in which great turbulence has been created by two inlets of air at different psi. The particles hit one another, and are removed by centrifugal means, collected in a cyclone setup or in a bag above the cyclone.

Such particles become highly electrically charged and during the operation, sparks are possible. This causes a danger of dust explosions, and micropulverization usually takes place in isolated, explosion-proof rooms. Due to the small particle size, the micronized powders also become very cohesive.

Special handling techniques in blending are, therefore, necessary in order to separate the small particles. (Otherwise they would simply behave as particles as large as the agglomerates they form.) This is one reason for employing intensifier bars in V-blenders and/or using other high-intensity mixers. In some cases (e.g., intrinsic factor), pyrogenic silica is used to keep the cohesive or charged particles apart. If done on a small scale, screening must be carried out in order to get the small silica particles "in between" the cohesive drug particles.

4.5 PARTICLE SHAPE AND SIZE DEFINITIONS

When a powder is milled, one usually describes the comminution in terms of a particle size of the solid after milling. In other words, the fineness of the powder is characterized by a number, e.g., a diameter.

Particles, of course, will have different shapes, but for the sake of discussion we shall assume in the following that they are cubical, with a side length of d cm. At times we shall (more conventionally) assume them to be spherical, in which case d would be the diameter. The preference in using a cubical approximation is that this shape is to some degree realistic when it comes to crystalline materials. On the other hand, granulations are better approximated by a spherical particle shape. The problem arises that in characterizing fineness, one is making a series of approximations.

Figure 4.5 shows different ways of defining a diameter.

The "diameter" can be simply the longest or the shortest linear dimension of the crystal. If one can calculate the area of the particle, one may obtain

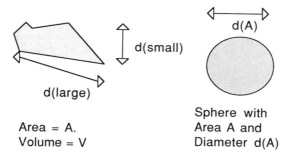

Area = A.
Volume = V

Sphere with
Area A and
Diameter d(A)

FIGURE 4.5. *Diameter definitions.*

the diameter, d_A, which is the diameter of a circle with the same area as the particle. This technique has been used microscopically.

Hence, d_A, the so-called area-mean diameter, is given by:

$$\pi d_A^2/4 = A \quad \text{or} \quad d_A = 2[A/\pi]^{1/2} \tag{4.8}$$

More conventional is the so-called surface mean diameter, which is the diameter of a sphere that has the same surface area as the particle. Noting that the surface area of a sphere is

$$\text{Area of sphere} = 4\pi r^2 = \pi d^2 \tag{4.9}$$

where r is the radius, the expression for this so-called single particle surface mean diameter becomes:

$$\pi d_s^2 = a \quad \text{or} \quad d_s = [a/\pi]^{1/2} \tag{4.10}$$

Small case a is used to designate the area of one single particle. (Large A will be used for the surface area of a powder sample.)

It will be seen later that there are instruments that can measure the volume of an odd-shaped particle, so by a definition similar to that shown in Figure 4.5, and noting that the volume of a sphere is:

$$v = (4/3)\pi r^3 = \pi d^3/6 \tag{4.11}$$

where small case v implies an individual particle. The expression for the so-called single particle volume mean diameter then becomes

$$v = \pi d_v^3/6 \quad \text{or} \quad d_v = [6v/\pi]^{1/3} \tag{4.12}$$

A concept frequently used is the concept of a shape factor, Γ. This is defined as the ratio between the area and the 2/3 power of the volume (which would then have units of cm²). For a single particle this would translate to:

$$a = \Gamma[v]^{2/3} \qquad (4.13)$$

This is exemplified for a cube of side d. The area, a, is six times the area of the side, so that:

$$a = 6d^2 \qquad (4.14)$$

The volume is d^3, so that the 2/3 power of the volume is:

$$v^{2/3} = d^2 \qquad (4.15)$$

Combination of Equations (4.13) to (4.15) then shows that for a cube, $\Gamma = 6$. The largest of all shape factors is for a sphere.

If, as in the above case, the shape factor is independent of the size of the particle, then the shape is called *isometric*. Examples of isometric shapes are a cube, a sphere, and a cylinder that is as high as it is wide.

4.6 NORMAL DISTRIBUTIONS

If all the particles in a sample are of the same size, then the powder is, as mentioned earlier, monodisperse. Only very few instances in technology produce this situation. (Ragweed pollen was used for many years as a calibrator for particle size instruments because it is quite monodisperse.) Fairly monodisperse products are products like cornstarch, which has a fairly narrow particle size distribution (25–35 μm). In this case the particles are also very spherical, so that the definition of its diameter or size follows naturally. Such very narrow distributions of powders approximate a so-called normal or Gaussian distribution.

Suppose a sample of twelve particles of cornstarch were measured somehow [13] and the results in Table 4.1 were obtained.

To convert these numbers into frequencies, it is noted that there are twelve particles in total, i.e., dividing each number by 12 will give the frequency or multiplying this by 100 will give the percentage frequency. This is done in Table 4.2.

The numbers should, of course, add up to 1.00 and 100%. The reason they do not is that the first, third, and last row entries are rounded off. It is conventional, in such cases, to adjust the largest numeral (in this case 0.333

TABLE 4.1 Particle Sizes of a Sample (of 12 Particles) of Cornstarch.

Particle Size Range	Number of Occurrences
25–27	1
27–29	3
29–31	4
31–33	3
33–35	1

or 33.3%) by an amount that will make the total become 1.00 (or 100%). This is, of course, only allowable when adjustment for rounding-off errors is made. (For instance, if the total had been 0.92 or 92%, then a systematic error would certainly have occurred.)

If the frequency is plotted as a function of the midpoint of the diameter ranges, then a plot as shown in Figure 4.6 results. This is denoted a *frequency histogram*.

It is noted in the table that all the intervals are of the same lengths (i.e., have the same statistical weight), and the frequencies can, therefore, be plotted as a curve. This has been shown in Figure 4.7. Such plots are called *frequency plots*.

The average and the standard deviation of the numbers in Table 4.1 are found as follows: the average is, of course

$$d_{avg} = \frac{1 \times 26 + 3 \times 28 + 4 \times 30 + 3 \times 32 + 1 \times 34}{1 + 3 + 4 + 3 + 1} \quad (4.16)$$

Symbolically this is written:

$$d_{avg} = \Sigma(nd)/\Sigma n \quad (4.17)$$

and is the number average mean diameter or the arithmetic mean diameter.

TABLE 4.2 Particle Sizes of a Sample (of 12 Particles) of Cornstarch.

Particle Size Range (μm)	Number of Occurrences (n)	Fractional Frequency	Percent Frequency
25–27	1	0.083	8.3%
27–29	3	0.25	25.0%
29–31	4	0.333 (0.334)	33.3% (33.4%)
31–33	3	0.25	25%
33–35	1	0.083	8.3%
Totals	12	0.999 (1.00)	99.9% (100%)

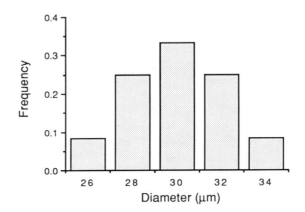

FIGURE 4.6. *Frequency histogram of particles in Table 4.1.*

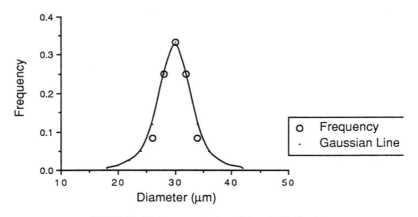

FIGURE 4.7. *Frequency plot of data in Table 4.1.*

The variance of a data set of n numbers is given by the formula:

$$s^2 = [\Sigma(x - x_{avg})]^2/(n - 1) \tag{4.18}$$

i.e., the "sum of squares"

$$ss = [\Sigma(x - x_{avg})]^2 \tag{4.19}$$

divided by $(n - 1)$, the degrees of freedom.

For computational purposes it is often more convenient to use an expression for the sum of squares which is completely equal to Equation (4.19) and is:

$$ss = \Sigma(x^2) - \{[\Sigma(x)]^2/n\} \tag{4.20}$$

since this latter expression does not involve first calculating the average or mean, x_{avg}.

The standard deviation is then the square root of the variance.

$$s = \{[\Sigma(x - x_{avg})]^2/(n - 1)\}^{1/2} \tag{4.21}$$

The standard deviation for the data in Tables 4.1 and 4.2 is given as shown in Table 4.3.

Hence the standard deviation is

$$s = [56/(12 - 1)]^{1/2} = 2.26$$

It is noted that the inflection point in the curve in Figure 4.7 occurs at $30 - 2.26 = 27.74$ and at $30 + 2.26 = 32.26$ μm. Some degree of normalization of the curve can be obtained by adjusting the mean to zero, and

TABLE 4.3 Standard Deviation of Data in Table 4.1 (x_{avg} = 30).

Diameter* (μm)	$x - x_{avg}$	n	$n(x - x_{avg})^2$	$(x - x_{avg})/s$
26	−4	1	16	−2.09
28	−2	3	12	−1.05
30	0	4	0	0
32	2	3	12	1.05
34	4	1	16	2.09
Total	0		56	

*These numbers are the midpoints of the intervals in Table 4.2.

by making the abscissa in units of standard deviations. This latter is accomplished in the last column of Table 4.3. This results in the curve in Figure 4.8.

If the normal deviate is denoted

$$z_1 = (x - x_{avg})/s$$

then this is an estimate of

$$z = (x - \mu)/\sigma \qquad (4.22)$$

where μ and σ are the true mean and standard deviation of the entire population from which the sample (of twelve particles) was taken.

The Gaussian frequency curve is represented by:

$$y = (2\pi)^{-1/2} \exp(z^2/2) \qquad (4.23)$$

This is the curve (not the points) shown in Figures 4.7 and 4.8.

If we ask ourselves, finally, what fraction (or what percentage) of particles are below 29 μm, we then see that four particles (or a fraction of $4/12 = 0.333$ or $0.083 + 0.25$) are below the given particle diameter. This calculation is carried out for the data in Table 4.1 in Table 4.4.

It is noted that for the non-cumulative curve, the midpoints of the intervals are used, but for the cumulative curve the interval endpoint is used. When plotted in the fashion shown here, it is referred to as an undersize dis-

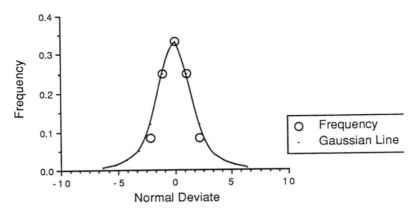

FIGURE 4.8. Normal error curve (frequency curve).

TABLE 4.4 Cumulative Numbers for the Data in Tables 4.1–4.3.

Particle Size Range (μm)	Largest Particle (d')	Fractional Frequency	Percent Frequency	Cumulative Frequency < d'	Cumulative % < d'
25–27	27	0.083	8.3%	0.083	8.3%
27–29	29	0.25	25.0%	0.333	33.3%
29–31	31	0.334	33.4%	0.667	66.7%
31–33	33	0.25	25%	0.917	91.7%
33–35	35	0.083	8.3%	1.0	100%

tribution curve. The opposite could, of course, have been done, i.e., one would pose the question: What is the fraction or percent of particles above a given particle size? In that case, the lower limit of each interval would be used.

If the data in the last column of Table 4.4 is plotted versus the first, then the data in Figure 4.9 results, and it is seen that an S-shaped distribution curve results.

Probability paper is a type of paper that straightens out this type of S-shaped curve. An example of probability paper is shown in Figure 4.10. The right-hand scale is the one used.

If the data in the last column of Table 4.4 are plotted as "Percent Smaller Than" the diameter in column 2 on probability paper, then the graph becomes a straight line. This is shown in Figure 4.11.

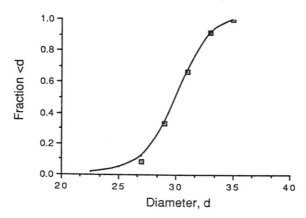

FIGURE 4.9. *Cumulative frequency curve (normal distribution curve).*

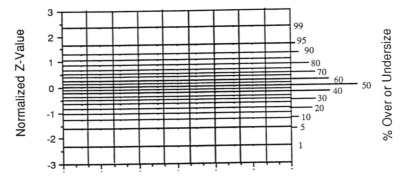

FIGURE 4.10. Probability paper.

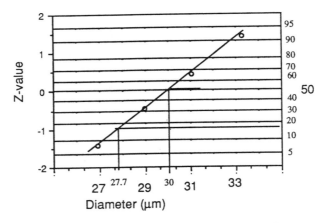

FIGURE 4.11. Data from Table 4.4 plotted on probability paper.

It is noted that at 50% the abscissa value is the average (mean).[3] If the *x*-value at 16% is noted, and subtracted from the mean, then the standard deviation results.

Particle sizes of milled powders [14,15] are usually log-normal, i.e., if the frequency is plotted versus log [*d*], then a straight line results. This will be covered in Chapter 14. Granulations, on the other hand, are frequently normally distributed [15].

4.7 REFERENCES

1. Berry, C. E. 1946. *Ind. Eng. Chem.*, 38:672.
2. Nakai, Y., S. Nakajima, K. Yamamota, K. Terada and T. Konno. 1980. *Chem. Pharm. Bull.*, 28:652.
3. Nakai, E., S. Fukuoka, S. Nakajima and K. Yamamoto. 1977. *Chem. Pharm. Bull.*, 25:96, 2490, 3340.
4. Nakai, Y., E. Fukuoka, S. Nakajima and Y. Iida. *Chem. Pharm. Bull.*, 25:2983, 3419.
5. Hatcher, W. J. and L. Y. Sadler. 1975. *J. Catalysis*, 38:73.
6. Goujon, G. and Mutaftshchier. 1976. *J. Colloid and Interface Sci.*, 57:148.
7. Yamaguchi, G. and K. Sakamoto. 1959. *Bull. Chem. Soc. Japan*, 32:1364.
8. Pearce, C. E. and D. Lewis. 1972. *J. Catalysis*, 26:318.
9. Parrott, E. G. 1986. *The Theory and Practice of Industrial Pharmacy, Third Edition*, H. A. Lieberman, L. Lachman, J. L. Koenig, eds., Philadelphia, PA: Lea and Febiger, p. 21 ff.
10. Carstensen, J. T., F. Puisieux, A. Mehta and M. A. Zoglio. 1978. *Int. J. Pharm.*, 1:65.
11. Mehta, A., K. Adams, M. A. Zoglio and J. T. Carstensen. 1977. *J. Pharm. Sci.*, 66:1462.
12. Carstensen, J. T. 1973. *Theory of Pharmaceutical Systems, Vol. 2*. New York, NY: Acad. Press, p. 238.
13. Carstensen, J. T. 1977. *Pharmaceutics of Solids and Solid Dosage Forms*. New York, NY: Wiley, p. 48.
14. Carstensen, J. T. and M. Patel. 1974. *J. Pharm. Sci.*, 63:1494.
15. Steiner, G., M. Patel and J. T. Carstensen. 1974. *J. Pharm. Sci.*, 63:1395.

4.8 PROBLEMS (CHAPTER 4)*

(1) A monodisperse powder with a diameter of 500 μm is milled to an average particle size of 50 μm. In a second experiment the same powder

---

[3]Actually the median, but for fairly large data the difference between median and mean is small.

*Answers on page 237.

is milled to an average particle size of 5 μm. What is the ratio of energy consumption for the two millings?

(2) 100 g 20 mesh powder is milled for 5 minutes in a ball mill and then sieved through a 20 mesh screen. 90 grams is retained on the screen. How much would be expected to be retained after 10 minutes? (Consider the times "short.")

CHAPTER 5

Tablets

By far the most common dosage form is a tablet. A tablet is a solid body that has been formed by placing it in a cavity, and applying sufficient pressure to it so "it hangs together." The reason for this happening will be discussed in the following.

5.1 PILLS

Historically, the first "formed" dosage form was a pill. In pill-making, drug is added to a doughy mixture of triglycerides, and rolled into a long snake-like form; this is then cut into pieces and rolled, and the spherical body formed is a pill. There are machines that make pills, but pills are so uncommon nowadays as to be essentially extinct. The problems with pills are (1) that they cannot (even when the process is mechanized) be made at a very high rate, (2) the doughy excipients used are such that they often impair the bioavailability of the drug substance, and (3) they have marginal content uniformity partly due to difficulty of mixing, and partly due to weight variation.

The word "pill" persists in the lay, but tablets are what are commonly prescribed, and professionally they should be referred to as such. The word "pill" with the prefixed article "the" has been made by the press into a synonym for oral contraceptives. It would be a bit much to expect that it be correctly referred to as "the tablet," so in that sense the word "pill" still stays in usage.

5.2 SINGLE PUNCH TABLET MACHINES (ECCENTRIC MACHINES)

The manner in which tablets are made is exemplified in Figure 5.1 by the operational steps of a single punch tablet machine (Stokes E or F). The

63

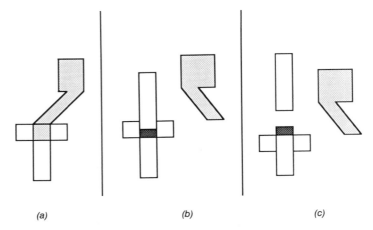

FIGURE 5.1. *One-sided tableting (single punch machine): (a) die fills; (b) upper punch compresses; and (c) punches rise, expel tablet.*

powder flows from the hopper (the shoe) into the die cavity, the bottom of which consists of the lower (movable) punch. The shoe then moves back, and the upper punch comes down and compresses the powder into a tablet. Both punches then move up and the tablet is ejected. The shoe then moves in over the punch again, knocking the tablet away, the lower punch drops into its lowest position, and the cycle repeats. If the lowest position of the lower punch is raised, then less powder flows into the die cavity, hence the "fill weight" is decreased. In this manner it is possible to control the weight of a tablet. The lower the lowest position of the upper punch, the harder the tablet will become. The hardness is determined with a hardness tester and the dimensions of the tablet are determined with a caliper or micrometer. There is a limit to how hard a tablet can be compressed, since if the upper punch position is too low, then the machine will freeze up.

In large scale, tablets are made on rotary machines (Figure 5.2). It is seen that the punches ride on cams, so that they are in a particular position at a given stage of the rotation. By the pressure wheels (where the tablet is formed), the top punch is in its lowest position, for instance.

Figure 5.3 shows the side view while Figure 5.4 gives the top view of the die table and detail view of the feedframe. The powder enters from the hopper to the feedframe, and from here it feeds into the cylindrical die cavity, created by the bottom position of the lower punch and the walls of the die. At the last part of the stage below the feedframe, the lower punch raises a bit, so that the die is full, and can be scraped clean at the end of the feed-

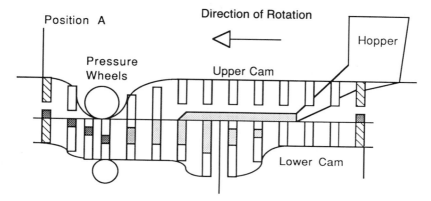

FIGURE 5.2. *Side view schematic of rotary machine. The two cross-hatched punches are the same, i.e., the movement has come full cycle.*

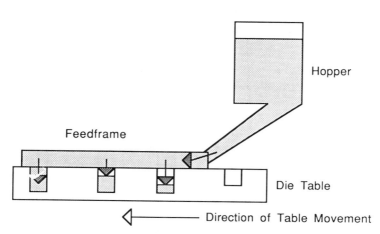

FIGURE 5.3. *Hopper and feedframe in a rotary machine.*

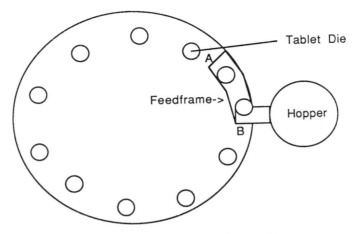

FIGURE 5.4. *Die table on a rotary machine.*

frame. (After that, on some machines, it is lowered a bit again.) The top
punch then comes down and the bottom punch up, and the tablet is compressed from both sides. Then both punches rise and the tablet is ejected.
This is position A in the right of Figure 5.2, which is also the cross-hatched
punch at the left. The ejected tablet is knocked off by a knock-off bar at the
back of the feedframe, and the cycle repeats.

5.3 BOND FORMATION IN TABLETS

If a solid body [Figure 5.5(a)] is subjected to a force, then it will first
elastically deform [Figure 5.5(b)]. At this stage, if the force is removed,
then the body will return to its original state. The force divided by the surface area is called the stress (in this case compressive stress). By application of the force (stress), the dimensions change, and the magnitude of the
dimensional change is called the strain. These dimensional changes can be
defined in several ways, one of which is to consider the relative change in
volume, $\Delta V/V$.

Example 5.1

A force of 1 kN (kiloNewton) is applied to a solid cube of a solid. The
original volume is 1.00 cm^3 and after application of the force the height of
the cube has decreased to 0.9 cm, whereas the (two) base dimension(s) have
increased to 1.02 cm. What is the relative volume strain?

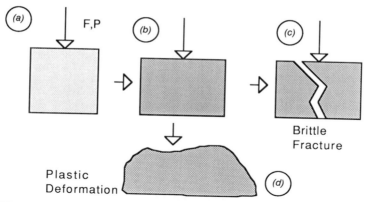

FIGURE 5.5. *Changes in shape on failure of a solid particle under stress. (Please note that the squares do not represent tablets, but rather particles in a tablet.)*

Answer 5.1

The new volume is $0.9 \times 1.02 \times 1.02 = 0.936$, so $\Delta V = 0.064$ cm, i.e., the strain is $0.064/1.000 = 6.4\%$ or 0.064.

The stages (c) and (d) in Figure 5.5 are denoted the elastic limit. Beyond this limit there is either breakage or flow, and the situations are referred to as brittle fracture or plastic deformation respectively. The critical value can be expressed either as a force (E, measured in several different force units: Newton, kg force, kN, dyne) or a stress (ϕ, measured in several different units of force per area: Pascal, kg/cm^2, lb/sq. inch). The linear portion in Figure 5.6 is denoted Hooke's law, i.e., the strain is proportional to the stress.

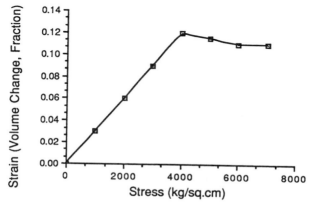

FIGURE 5.6. *Stress-strain diagram for a block of solid.*

In a tablet press it is necessary to exceed the elastic limit before bonds are formed in the tablet.[4] Bond formation starts when the elastic limit is exceeded. The number of bonds formed, N_f, are proportional to the amount of pressure (stress) exerted during the downstroke of the upper punch.

It is important to know which of the two "breaking" modes of the particles happens in tablets. A given substance (e.g., sulfanilamide) may fail in brittle fracture, another substance (e.g., sodium chloride) may fail in plastic deformation. At times, both occur to some degree, and in a tablet containing many substances (drugs and excipients) some may bond one way, some another.

In the early development of tablet physics, investigators were interested in how the particle size changed as compression pressure was increased, and Higuchi and Busse [1–3] at Wisconsin, studying sodium chloride, found the surface area to decrease, whereas Shotton [4,5] in England studying sulfanilamide, found it to increase. It is apparent (and logical) that when plastic deformation occurs, the bonding occurs by particles flowing together, and the bonds represent area lost, whereas the opposite is true in brittle fracture, where smaller particles, i.e., larger surface areas, are created.

The type of bonding is also important in formula decisions. Bonding is impaired by lubricants[5] in plastic deformation: the magnesium stearate becomes fluid under pressure and gets in between the surfaces of the particles, and the common surfaces cannot get close enough together to bond.[6] Hydroxyapatite (Tritab) bonds in this fashion, and magnesium stearate in concentrations above 1% makes it impossible to make a good tablet. Dicalcium phosphate (A-tab, Ditab), however, bonds by brittle fracture, and can sustain very high levels of lubricant (above 5%).[7]

---

[4]The famous English pharmaceuticist, E. T. Shotton, recalled at one time, that he got started in tablet physics, because a friend of his, a polymer chemist, had trouble making a resin of large enough particle size. He suggested tableting it, but to his surprise was not able to. The powder that had flowed into the die simply was ejected unchanged, i.e., the elastic limit was very high for the substance, and was not exceeded in the press.

[5]Lubricants will be discussed shortly, and their function is to aid in the ejection of the material from the punch after compression of the tablet. Magnesium stearate is the most common lubricant.

[6]In the compression, the bond is formed when two molecules in neighboring crystals or particles arrive at a proximity that is close to a molecular lattice spacing (i.e., of an order of magnitude of Angstroms). Then molecular forces become effective. These are inversely proportional to a higher power of the distance between centers, and one function of the compression is to bring molecules from neighboring particles that close together.

[7]Levels of magnesium stearate above 1% are usually not needed and not advocated, as will be touched on at a later point.

5.4 COMPRESSION PROFILES

In the early 1950s, Professors Higuchi and Busse at the School of Pharmacy, U.W., developed the first instrumented tablet machine. By means of strain gauges, they were able to monitor the force sensed by (1) the upper punch, (2) the lower punch, and (3) the die wall, during the compression cycle. A characteristic cycle profile is shown in Figure 5.7.

Point A corresponds to the elastic limit, point B the point where the pressure on the upper punch is discontinued. At this point there is a "pull" on the tablet surface (much like a corkscrew), and at C the effect of the upper punch on the tablet ceases, and the tablet simply expands by itself. The reason that there is a pressure (stress) sensed between B and C is that the tablet expands more rapidly than the punch moves back, hence there is tension between them.

The cycle ends at point D, and the ordinate (OD) at this point is the residual die wall pressure. To eject the tablet it is now necessary to overcome this force. Figure 5.8 diagrams this situation, and it is noted that it is similar to the frictional scheme diagram in Figure 2.8 in Chapter 2. The normal force is, here, the residual die wall force, and the ejection force is the tangential force (Figure 5.8). By making tablets at different applied pressures, one obtains different residual die wall forces and different ejection forces, and it can be observed that the ejection force is (often[8]) proportional to the residual die wall force:

$$E = \mu D \tag{5.1}$$

It is obvious that it is advantageous to reduce the ejection force, and hence a lubricant is added to the tablet formulation. The most common lubricant is magnesium stearate in the amount of 0.5%–1%. Beyond a certain percentage there is no advantage in further addition of magnesium stearate (or other lubricant [6]). The amount of lubricant used is a balancing situation, because enough has to be added to assure good ejection, but the lubricant affects dissolution adversely. In some cases, as discussed under bond formation, the lubricant also affects the bond strength [7]. Formulators therefore often optimize the amount of lubricant used by statistical means [8].

In the amounts used, enough magnesium stearate is squeezed out to the die wall/tablet interface, so that the ejection force is sufficiently reduced to allow stress-free ejection.

The magnesium stearate serves another purpose as well. It is assumed in

---

[8]For the friction concept to work, the surfaces must be independent of applied load. This is not quite true, for instance, if brittle fracture occurs.

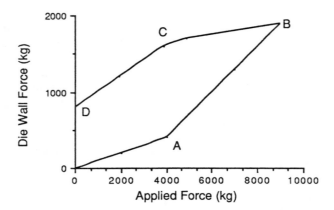

FIGURE 5.7. *Compression cycle.*

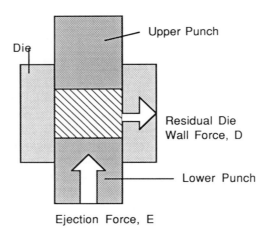

FIGURE 5.8. *Residual die wall force, D, and ejection force, E.*

the previous paragraphs that the process by which the compression act progresses is as follows.

(1) The powder flows into the die cavity and attains, immediately, a loose configuration (cascaded apparent density).

(2) As the upper punch comes down, it attains its closest packing.

(3) As the punch comes down even further, the particles have no place "to go" anymore, and start distorting. In the first phase of this the distortion is elastic, and if the pressure is released at this point, no tablet will have been formed.

(4) Once the elastic limit is reached the bonding will start, until the dead point (the lowest point of the upper punch) has been reached.

(5) As the upper punch is released there is a stress (uniaxial expansion) which occurs in the tablet.

(6) The punches now ascend, and there is friction between the tablet and the die wall.

(7) The tablet is completely ejected. In many cases [9] there is an expansion of the tablet as it comes out of the die. It is often not possible to put the tablet back into the die after it is ejected.

The above sequence may well be the course of action in a single punch machine, but in high-speed machines, the closest packing may not be reached in some areas of the tablet before compression starts in another part of it. Tablets made on a high-speed machine will (almost) always, at the same compression pressure, have a higher porosity than those made on a slow machine (or a stationary, hydraulic press).

The tablets produced will have different apparent densities in various parts of the tablet, due to these phenomena, and it is desirable to minimize this. Magnesium stearate (and other lubricants) acts as a glidant in the die so that the particles more easily rearrange, and in this manner it aids in the making of high-quality tablets.

This effect of the magnesium stearate is best illustrated by the so-called Higuchi R-ratio [10,11] which is the ratio between the upper and the lower punch forces. This should be close to unity for good particle flow in the die.

5.5 THICKNESS (POROSITY) OF A TABLET

In general, as a rule, the higher the compression pressure, the thinner the tablet will become. We shall see shortly that this is true only up to a certain limit.

TABLE 5.1 Porosity as a Function of Applied Pressure for a Powder with True Density 1.25 g/cm² and Employing a Tablet Weight of 375 mg and a Punch with a 1 cm² Cross-Sectional Area.

Applied Pressure, kP	Thickness cm	Porosity	− ln [Porosity]
2,000	1.2	0.4	0.916
2,500	0.65	0.5	0.693
3,000	0.42	0.286	1.253
4,000	0.34	0.118	2.140
5,000	0.32	0.062	2.773
6,000	0.31	0.032	3.442
7,000	0.305	0.016	4.135
(8,000)	(0.300)	0	

Table 5.1 shows the tablet thickness as a function of the maximum applied force in a tablet operation.

These data are plotted in Figure 5.9 as thickness versus applied pressure. The tablet cannot become thinner[9] than what corresponds to its true density. (In this case the porosity is zero.) Here this value corresponds to a tablet thickness of 0.3 cm.

Example 5.2

What is the smallest thickness, h_∞, of the tablet in Table 5.1?

Answer 5.2

The volume of the solid in the tablet is

$$0.375/1.25 = 0.3 \text{ cm}^3$$

If there is no porosity, then this volume equals the height, h_∞, times the cross-sectional area (1.00 cm²), i.e.:

$$h_\infty \times 1.00 = 0.3, \quad \text{i.e.,} \quad h_\infty = 0.3 \text{ cm}$$

as shown in the table.

[9]It is, theoretically, possible to compress further than this point, since non-porous solids may be compressed further. This may possibly happen in a tablet machine although it is usually only experienced at very high pressures.

Example 5.3

Calculate the porosity of a tablet compressed at 3,000 kP.

Answer 5.3

This can be done by calculating the apparent density and knowing the true density. A bit easier is to note that the void space is $(0.42 - 0.3) = 0.12$ cm³ and the total space is 0.42 cm³, so that

$$\epsilon = 0.12/0.42 = 0.286$$

If instead of thickness, the negative of the natural logarithm[10] of the porosity is plotted versus applied pressure, then the data linearize as shown in Figure 5.10. Such a plot is called an Athy-Heckel (or simply a Heckel) plot [12–16]. The slope of the plot is $1/(3\phi)$ where ϕ is the yield value (elastic limit).

Example 5.4

In Figures 5.9 and 5.10, what is the average elastic limit of the material? The cross-sectional area of the tablet is 1 cm².

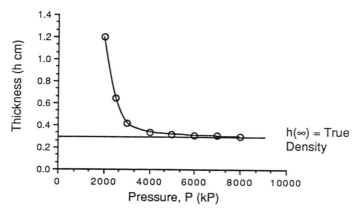

FIGURE 5.9. *Data in Table 5.1 plotted linearly.*

[10]It is strictly an arbitrary convention in literature to plot $-\ln [\epsilon]$ rather than $\ln [\epsilon]$. If the latter were done, then the data would still be linear, but with a negative slope.

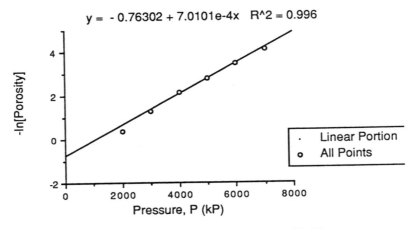

FIGURE 5.10. *Heckel plot of data in Table 5.1.*

Answer 5.4

The slope of the line is 0.0007, so that $1/(3\phi) = 0.0007$, i.e., $\phi = 1428/3 = 476 \text{ kP} = 476 \text{ kP/cm}^2$, the last equality because the cross-sectional area is 1 cm².

There are cases where, if the compression pressure (maximum applied pressure) is elevated sufficiently, the thickness will start to increase as the pressure is increased. Examination of the tablets formed in this region will reveal that they have hairline cracks on the walls, so that the expansion (BCD in Figure 5.17) has broken the tablet bonds completely in certain areas. This of course makes the tablet thicker than if the cracks were not there.

Worse still, if this type of behavior starts occurring at relatively low compression pressures, the tablet can "cap." This means that the hairline crack has propagated all the way through the tablet, which then falls apart in two pieces. This usually happens close to the crown, as shown in Figure 5.11.

5.6 HARDNESS OF TABLETS

The hardness of a tablet is a function of how much pressure has been exerted in making it. Figure 5.12 shows a typical hardness/pressure graph. At high pressures the tablet will start to cap, and the hardness will go down again. A capped tablet is shown in Figure 5.11, and is a common type of defect. The reason for it occurring is that when the upper punch starts "go-

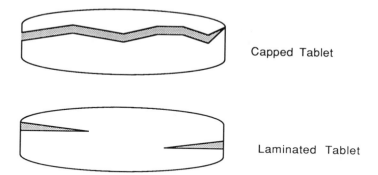

Capped Tablet

Laminated Tablet

FIGURE 5.11. *Capped tablet and laminated tablet.*

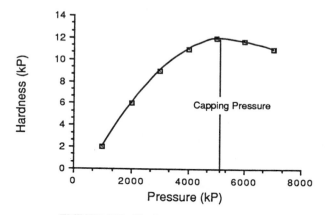

FIGURE 5.12. *Hardness/pressure diagram.*

ing up" again, the pressure is released, and the tablet can expand in only one direction (uniaxial expansion). This causes stress on the tablet, and although the applied pressure makes the tablet stronger, at a given point the extra strength acquired by the additional tableting pressure is offset by the additional stress in the expansion.

It was seen earlier that during the compression a number of bonds, N_f, are formed, and the number of bonds is proportional to the applied pressure. If the pressure is doubled, then the number of bonds are doubled, i.e.

$$N_f = \beta P \qquad (5.2)$$

However, when the upper punch is removed a number of bonds, N_d, are destroyed, and this number is proportional to a power of P, e.g., to P^2, i.e.

$$N_d = \phi P^2 \qquad (5.3)$$

Hence the total number of bonds in the ejected tablet will be:

$$N = N_f - N_d = \beta P - \phi P^2 \qquad (5.4)$$

This is a parabola with a maximum at:

$$dN/dP = 0 = \beta - 2\phi P, \text{ i.e., it occurs at } P = \beta/(\phi 2) \qquad (5.5)$$

as shown in Figure 5.12.

5.7 CLASSIFICATION OF MATERIALS REGARDING COMPRESSION PROPERTIES

To make a tablet of a substance, it must, first of all, compress at pressures that are obtainable on the tablet press, i.e., the yield value must be low. Furthermore it must flow well enough, so that the cavity formed by the die and the lower punch is filled up with powder by the time it is compressed.

Flow rates will be covered separately later in this chapter, suffice it to say at this point that flow rates are a function of particle size and shape. In general the larger the particle (up to a limit) and the more spherical it is, the more rapidly it will flow into a die cavity.

To compress a powder, then, the situations shown in Table 5.2 apply.

TABLE 5.2 Types of Preparation for Tablet Making.

Compressibility	Flow	Action
Good	Good	Directly Compressible
Good	Poor	Roller Compact
		Slug
		Wet Granulate
Poor	Poor	Wet Granulate
Poor	Good	Wet Granulate

5.8 DIRECT COMPRESSION

There are several direct compression excipients available on the market.

- A-tab: dibasic calcium phosphate anhydrate
- Ditab: dibasic calcium phosphate dihydrate
- Tritab: hydroxyapatite
- Avicel: microcrystalline cellulose
- Lactoses: spray-dried (monohydrate, partly amorphous), DC grade (anhydrous), and Tablettose™ (granulated)

In all of the above cases, if a drug is present in an amount of less than 16%, then the characteristics of the powder are usually those of the directly compressible excipient.

It is often desirable to directly compress rather than wet granulate. In the latter procedure, one adds water, then uses energy to remove it again, so that energy-wise it is not economical. Wet granulation is advantageous in some respects, however, and these will be brought out in the following.

But often, formulation decisions are made based on the choice between the two routes: wet or dry. If a poorly compressible drug is to be given in a 50 mg dose, then it is possible to make a 100 mg tablet by wet route but not one by direct compression. But there is nothing magic about a small tablet, and if a tablet of size $50/0.16 = 312$ mg or more were made, then direct-compressed tablets would be feasible.

Some of the direct compression excipients contain calcium and phosphorus, and are excellent for food supplement (multivitamin + mineral tablets) in that the excipient is, at the same time, an active ingredient.

5.9 SIZE AND IDENTIFICATION OF TABLETS

The size of a tablet is the first property to decide, once it is decided in product development what the strengths should be (e.g., 5, 10, and 25 mg).

Aside from the compression approach alluded to above, there are several factors that enter into the selection of the size of a tablet. It is desirable to have the tablet be distinct, so that it can be discerned from other medicaments, and this can be done by varying shape, color, size and of course by imprint. The importance of this cannot be overemphasized. For instance, Coumadin 2 mg tablets used to be peach-colored and the 5 mg tablets orange. Although the tablets were engraved with a 2 and a 5 respectively, they were hard to distinguish, and there was a host of lawsuits resulting from misprescriptions. The color of the 2 mg tablet was finally changed to green.[11]

Most tablets are standard convex, or flat-faced beveled.

5.10 POWDER FLOW REQUIREMENTS FOR TABLET GRANULATIONS

The quality of a product is partly the fact that each dosage unit (in this case each tablet) pretty much contains the amount of material that is claimed on the label. This has been alluded to previously (see Chapter 2), and in the case of a tablet, the content uniformity is a function of both the weight uniformity and of the uniformity of the mixture of whch the tablet is made. The USP test used to assess this is as follows.

It is apparent from the preceding that no individual tablet contains the "correct" amount of drug, but that there is a spread in the assays. It is necessary that the average of the tablets in a batch be close to the theoretical average. But the variation from tablet to tablet could be large. This could be due to three factors:

(1) The weights of all the tablets are not quite equal, e.g., they could range from 245 to 255 mg. The question is, how much variation should be allowed?

(2) The powder or granulation from which the tablet was made might not be quite uniform.

(3) On storage: the average of the tablet might have decreased in time.

There are regulations governing the effect of points 1 and 2 (and 3 as well). These are spelled out in the USP. The USP is issued every five years.

---

[11]It is interesting that (to the author's knowledge) the change was initiated by reasons other than attempts to more clearly distinguish between the colors (e.g., decertification of dye). In essence, the company is not responsible for misprescriptions, but lawsuits started after the color change had been made, because patients who had had doses larger than the ones prescribed by the physician, and who had suffered from it, started suing the company, claiming that the change in color showed that the company had originally been negligent.

The recent edition is the 1990 issue (USP XXII). The manner in which items are included in the USP is governed by the Revision Committee. Most of the drug entities in the USP are drugs whose patents have expired, and are, hence, the drugs that would be present as generic drugs.

5.10.1 Weight Variation and Content Uniformity (USP XXI, p. 1277)

USP XXI, p. 1277 states that

(1) Thirty tablets should be sampled, and ten selected.
(2) These ten tablets are assayed. An example of such assays is shown in Table 5.3.

The standard deviation of lot 1 is 0.319 and the average is 10.05. The relative standard deviation is

$$100 \times 0.319/10.05 = 3.15\% = 3\%$$

The USP requirements are that the batch is satisfactory if each of the tablet assays are larger than 85% of label claim (i.e., 8.5 mg) and smaller than 115% label claim (i.e., 11.5 mg). The relative standard deviation must be less than 6%. It is seen that these criteria are met with lot 1.

With lot 2, this is not the case:

- average = 10.5
- relative standard deviation = 7.1%
- first assay: below 8.5 mg

In such a case, the remaining twenty tablets are assayed. The mean and

TABLE 5.3 Content Uniformity.

Tablet#	Assay of Lot 1 (10 mg LC)	Assay of Lot 2 (10 mg LC)
1	9.8	8.4
2	10.2	10.2
3	10.1	10.1
4	9.7	11.1
5	10.2	10.2
6	9.9	9.9
7	9.5	9.5
8	10.4	10.4
9	10.2	10.2
10	10.5	10.5

standard deviation of the now thirty tablets are determined, and the RSD must be no higher than 7.8%, only one of the thirty tablets must be outside the 85/115% label claim bracket, and the outlier must be above 75 and less than 125% LC.

A single punch machine produces about sixty tablets per minute. If the tablet weight is 500 mg (0.5 g), then $0.5 \times 60 = 30$ g of material must flow through the hopper into the die per minute (or 0.5 g/sec). This is termed the required flow rate for the particular machine.

On a rotary machine there are two critical criteria: (1) the rate at which the powder flows from the hopper into the feedframe (W_1 g/sec), and (2) the rate at which it flows from the feedframe into the die (W_2 g/sec).

If the radius of the die table is 50 cm, and if the rotational speed of the machine, Ω, is, e.g., 30 rpm, i.e., 0.5 rotation per second, and if the length, a, of the feedframe is 20 cm, then the linear speed of the die will be $2\pi r \times \Omega$, i.e., in this case $2(3.14)(50)(0.5) = 157$ cm/sec. The length of time the powder is in contact with the feedframe is, therefore:

$$t = a/\{2\pi r \times \Omega\} = 20/157 = 0.13 \text{ sec} \qquad (5.6)$$

If the required fill weight of the tablet is 650 mg, then the minimum flow rate that will ascertain this would be 0.65 g/0.13 sec or

$$W_2 = 5 \text{ g/sec} \qquad (5.7)$$

If there are sixteen dies in the die table, then, since the machine runs at 30 RPM, $30 \times 16 = 480$ tablets are made per minute or eight tablets per second. Hence the flow or powder from the hopper into the die table must be at least:

$$W = 8 \times 650 = 5.2 \text{ g/sec} \qquad (5.8)$$

in other words slightly higher. The two requirements are not mutually exclusive. It can be shown that the flow rate, W, is a function of the diameter, D, of the orifice through which the flow occurs by the relation:

$$W = \beta \times D^{2.5} \qquad (5.9)$$

where β for a given powder sample is a constant (depending on, among other parameters, the cohesion hence indirectly on the repose angle).

It is interesting to note that companies often like to make one granulation and then compress it at different fill weights (in different size tablet dies) to get different strengths of the product.

Example 5.5

A 10 mg tablet is to be made to 100 mg fill weight in a 1/4 " (0.25 ") size. It is known that the formula flows just fast enough so that a 25 mg tablet can be made by filling 250 mg of the granulation into, e.g., a 3/8 " (0.375 ") punch and die. The contact time between granulation in the feedframe and the dies is 0.1 sec.

Answer 5.5

The flow rate of the granulation in a 0.375 inch die is 250 mg/0.1 sec = 2500 mg/sec. Inserting this into Equation (5.7) gives:

$$2500 = \beta (0.375)^{2.5} = 0.0861\beta, \quad \text{i.e.,} \quad \beta = 2500/0.0861 = 29,031$$

Now applying this to the smaller die, Equation (5.7) gives:

$$W = 29,031 \times (0.25)^{2.5} = 907 \text{ mg/sec}$$

Since the contact time is 0.1 sec, only 91 mg (not 100 mg) would flow into the dies in the machine, i.e., the fill weight could not be obtained.

Example 5.6

What would be a remedy for the situation in Example 5.5?

Answer 5.6

To run the machine more slowly (which is not economical) or to attempt somehow to make the powder flow more rapidly.

5.11 POWDER FLOW

If a powder flows poorly, then some improvement can at times be attained by means of a so-called glidant. *Talc* is an example of a glidant. Often, however, this is not sufficient in itself to improve the flow sufficiently, and other means of flow improvement are necessary.

There are two main factors that affect powder flow: particle size and particle shape. The closer a particle is to spherical the better it flows [17]. Small particles are very cohesive, and hence do not flow well [18,19] and (as a whole) increasing the particle size will improve flow. Figure 5.13 shows flow rates of various mesh cuts of a powder through a 0.5 cm orifice.

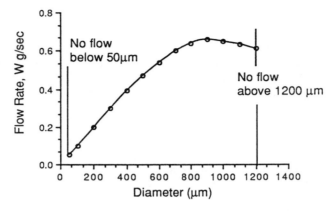

FIGURE 5.13. *Powder flow rates as a function of particle size.*

The reason there is no flow in the powder in Figure 5.13 below 50 μm is that the cohesive forces below this size become stronger than the gravitational force, and flow through the orifice is prevented. This, of course, is a function of the size of the orifice, and flow might be possible in a larger orifice.

It is obviously important to be able to calculate the cohesive stress, C [or the cohesive force, c (small case)]. To this end a Jenicke cell is used. Here powder is placed in two rings as shown in Figure 5.14. A load is placed on the powder in the top ring, and the force necessary to cause its displacement is made. Another weight is then utilized (usually one starts from the largest

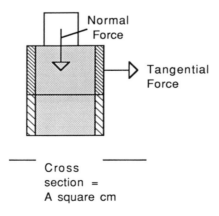

FIGURE 5.14. *Jenicke shear cell.*

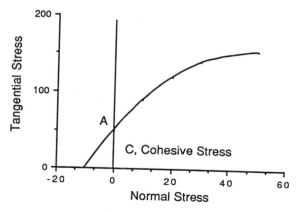

FIGURE 5.15. Jenicke locus.

weight and works downwards), and the tangential force measured, and so on until all the weights have been removed.

By so doing, a plot as shown in Figure 5.15 results, and the y-intercept (OA) of the plot is the cohesive stress, C.

The critical diameter, D, i.e., the diameter below which there is no flow, is tied into the cohesive stress in the following manner.

Assume flow through a tube of diameter D and of length h (Figure 5.16).

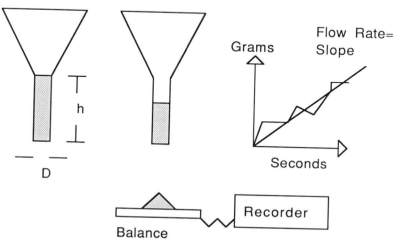

FIGURE 5.16. Powder in a tube, and recording flow rate determination.

Assume also that the apparent density in the tube is ϱ', so that the mass of the powder in the tube is:

$$m = (\pi D^2/4)\varrho' h \qquad (5.10)$$

The force in downwards direction is the gravitational force, i.e.

$$F_{down} = mg = g(\pi D^2/4)\varrho' h \qquad (5.11)$$

The force in the upwards direction is the cohesive stress times the area over which it works, i.e., the (inside) area of the cylinder. The area of a cylinder is the height times the circumference (πD)

$$F_{up} = C(\pi D)h \qquad (5.12)$$

Equating the two gives:

$$C(\pi D_{crit})h = g(\pi D_{crit}^2/4)\varrho' h \qquad (5.13)$$

where D_{crit} is the diameter below which there is no flow. This is solved to give:

$$D_{crit} = 4C/(gh\varrho') \qquad (5.14)$$

The regularity of flow is of importance as well. Often flow rates are measured by allowing the powder to flow out on a recording balance pan (Figure 5.16), and the grams on the pan as a function of time are recorded. This should be a straight line with a slope of W, the flow rate, but if the powder flows erratically, then the trace will be very irregular.

Particle size enlargement is effected by three means:

- slugging
- roller compaction
- wet granulation

It should be pointed out that particle size enlargement of the drug substance can be brought about by manipulation of the recrystallization step in the synthesis of the drug.

If a powder is compressible but does not flow well, then slugging may be employed. In slugging, tablets are made of the poorly flowing substance on a high-duty, slowly operating machine, into large dies. The dies are large so that the flow is sufficiently increased ($D^{2.5}$-dependence), but now the compression forces must be increased because the larger area dictates a larger force to attain a given pressure (the elastic limit being in stress units). When the slugs are gently milled, then the particles will be larger than prior to slugging, so that they will now flow sufficiently well to allow for compression into the appropriately smaller die dictated by the actual dosage form.

In roller compacting (Chillsonating), the powder is processed between two heavy duty rollers, compacted between the rolls, and emerges as a compressed sheet, which is then milled.

These two methods are necessary if the drug substance (e.g., aspirin) is sufficiently moisture sensitive, stability-wise, so it cannot be wet granulated. In cases where stability is not a moisture-dependent problem, wet granulation will be discussed next, and is a frequently used method of particle enlargement.

5.12 WORK AND ENERGY RELATIONS IN TABLET FORMATION

As the upper punch comes down, the pressure increases, and the work is force times the distance. The depth penetration of a punch can be gauged by means of displacement gauges during the compression, and a diagram such as shown in Figure 5.17 results [20–22]. The area ABD is the work transferred to the tablet during the compression, the cross-hatched area, CBD is the work lost during the uniaxial expansion of the tablet, and hence the work ABC is the energy that remains in the tablet, after it has expanded in the die.

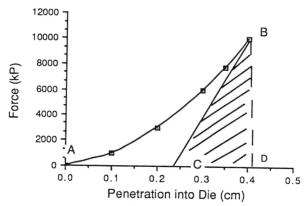

FIGURE 5.17. *Work diagram for a tablet.*

The smaller the cross-hatched area (elastic loss) the less the uniaxial stress upon decompression, i.e., the less will there be a tendency for the tablets to cap.

5.13 DISINTEGRATION OF TABLETS

It was recognized in the 1940s that tablets had to disintegrate in order for them to be bioavailable. In that period of time, the art and science of bio-pharmaceutics was not developed, primarily due to analytical limitations. Later, of course, in the 1950s and 1960s the pharmaceutical scientist became aware of the importance of dissolution rates as well. The general manner in which a tablet disintegrates is shown in Figure 5.18 and is as follows:

- The tablet wets down.
- Dissolution liquid penetrates the pore space.
- The disintegrant absorbs water and swells.
- This swelling causes the tablet to break down into granules.

These granules are NOT the same as the granules from which the tablet was made [23,24], and are the larger the more bonds have been formed, i.e., below the critical capping pressure, they are the larger, the higher the

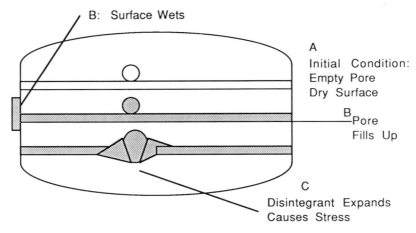

FIGURE 5.18. *Action of a disintegrant.*

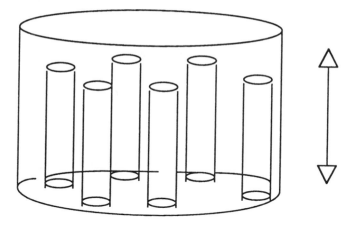

FIGURE 5.19. *USP disintegration apparatus.*

compression pressure. The actual pressure exerted by the disintegrant on the tablet has been determined instrumentally and follows the views stated previously [25].

Disintegration times are monitored routinely in tablet production using the apparatus shown in Figure 5.19.

The effect on disintegration times of increased tableting pressure (below the critical capping pressure) is as follows.

(1) At very low pressures the penetration of liquid into the tablet is virtually unhindered (almost like pouring water into a beaker) but the pores will be too large to allow the disintegrant swelling to cause stress. Hence, increase in compression pressure causes a larger and larger number of pores that have diameters less than the swollen disintegrant particle, and the disintegration time will decrease [26].

(2) Once the pores are sufficiently small, the penetration of the liquid into the disintegrant becomes the limiting step, and the disintegration time will increase on increasing pressure [27,28]. This is shown graphically in Figure 5.20.

Disintegrants and lubricants are added to wet granulated products after the granulation has been dried. The mixing time for the lubricant must be kept short because otherwise the lubricant may fluidize during the mixing step, and lose part of the lubricant properties that are necessary for flow in the tablet die.

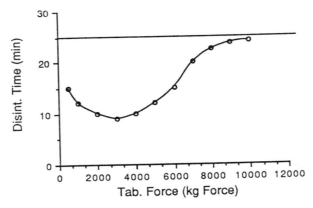

FIGURE 5.20. *Tablet disintegration as a function of applied tableting force.*

5.14 TABLET DISSOLUTION

When a tablet is exposed to dissolution, it must (1) wet, then (2) disintegrate. The particles that are formed are not prime particles, and water must then penetrate the granules before drug can diffuse out. The length of time, t_i, required for this is the lag time. The remainder of the curve becomes a diffusion type curve, i.e.

$$\ln [M/Mo] = -k\{t - t_i\} \tag{5.15}$$

k and t_i can be found from slope and intercept when the fraction not dissolved [M/Mo] is plotted versus time.

For example, the % data in Table 5.4 are obtained. The data are plotted linearly in Figure 5.21. It is noted from Figure 5.21 that the curve is slightly

TABLE 5.4 Dissolution Data of a Compressed Tablet.

Time	% Released	Fraction, [M/Mo] Not Released	ln [M/Mo]
6	9.5	0.905	−0.1
10	20	0.80	−0.22
15	33	0.67	−0.40
20	45	0.55	−0.59
40	70	0.30	−1.20
75	91	0.09	−2.40

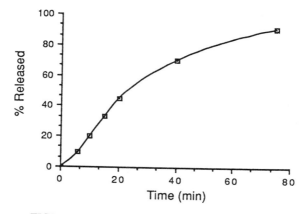

FIGURE 5.21. *Data from Table 5.4 plotted linearly.*

S-shaped. This is due to the lag time, where wetting, penetration, and disintegration take place.

The lag time is best obtained by plotting the data as ln [Fraction Undissolved] versus time, and this is shown in Figure 5.22.

The lag time is obtained as the point in time when ln $[M/Mo] = 0$ (i.e., all, theoretically, is undissolved), i.e.

$$0 = 0.098317 - 0.033435\ t_i \qquad (5.16)$$

or

$$t = 2.94 \text{ min} \qquad (5.17)$$

The disintegration time in the apparatus can be observed visually, and if this for instance were 1.5 min, then the time required for penetration and wetting would be $2.94 - 1.5 = 1.44$ min.

5.15 UNCOATED TABLET INGREDIENTS

It is seen from the above that the necessary ingredients for a wet granulated formula are as follows:

- drug (unless the product is a placebo in a clinical trial)
- filler (to attain the desired fill weight)
- binder (e.g., starch paste)

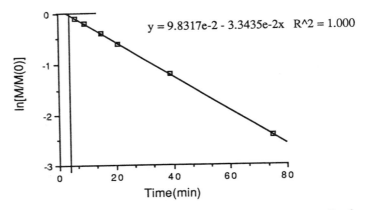

FIGURE 5.22. Dissolution data from Table 5.4 plotted as ln [fraction undissolved] versus time.

- disintegrant (e.g., crosspovidone or dry starch)
- glidant (e.g., talc)[12]
- lubricant (e.g., magnesium stearate)

There is an old pharmaceutical adage that insoluble drugs should be formulated with soluble fillers (e.g., lactose) and soluble drugs should be formulated with insoluble fillers (e.g., dicalcium phosphates). The reason for the former would seem logical from dissolution considerations, but it happens to be true in the latter case as well. If a soluble (particularly a very soluble) drug substance is formulated with, e.g., lactose, then, during the dissolution process, there is a tendency for gel formation about the drug particle, and this may hinder the dissolution.

5.16 REFERENCES

1. Higuchi, T., A. N. Rao, L. W. Busse and J. V. Swintosky. 1953. *J. Am. Pharm. Assoc.*, *Sci. Ed.*, 42:194.
2. Higuchi, T., E. Nelson and L. W. Busse. 1954. *J. Am. Pharm. Assoc.*, *Sci. Ed.*, 43:344.
3. Higuchi, T., L. N. Elowe and L. W. Busse. 1954. *J. Am. Pharm. Assoc.*, *Sci. Ed.*, 44:685.
4. Shotton, E. and D. Ganderton. 1960. *J. Pharm. Pharmacol*, 12:87T.
5. Shotton, E., J. J. Deer and D. Ganderton. 1963. *J. Pharm. Pharmacol*, 15:106T.
6. Fukomori, Y. and J. T. Carstensen. 1984. *Int. J. Pharm. Tech and Prod. Mfg.*, 4:1.

[12]Optional in tablets. Magnesium stearate is a good glidant in many systems.

7. Jarosz, P. J. and E. L. Parrot. 1984. *Drug Dev. and Ind. Pharm.*, 10.

8. Dawoodbhai, S., E. F. Suryanarayan, C. W. Woodruff and C. T. Rhodes. 1991. *Drug Dev. and Ind. Pharm.*, 17:1343.

9. Okutgen, M., M. Jordan, J. E. Hogan and M. E. Aulton. 1991. *Drug Dev. Ind. Pharm.*, 17:1177 and 1191.

10. Higuchi, T. 1954. *J. Am. Pharm. Assoc., Sci. Ed.*, 43:344.

11. Fessi, H., J.-P. Marty, F. Puisieux and J. T. Carstensen. 1986. *Int. J. Pharmaceutics*, 30:209.

12. Heckel, R. W. 1961. *Trans. Metal Soc. of AIME*, 221:671.

13. Athy, L. F. 1930. *Bull Am. Assoc. Petrol Geologist*, 14:1.

14. Carstensen, J. T., J.-M. Geoffroy, and C. Dellamonica. 1990. *Powder Techn.*, 62:119.

15. Yu, H. C. M., M. H. Rubinstein, I. M. Jackson and H. M. Elsabbagh. 1989. *Drug Dev. Ind. Pharm.*, 15:801.

16. Carstensen, J. T. and X.-P Hou. 1985. *Powder Technol.*, 42:153.

17. Ridgway, K. and R. Rupp. 1969. *J. Pharm. Pharmacol.*, 21:30T.

18. Carstensen, J. T. and P. L. Chan. 1977. *J. Pharm. Sci.*, 66:1235.

19. Jones, T. M. 1968. *J. Pharm. Sci.*, 57:2015.

20. Parmentier, W. 1974. Ph.D. thesis, Technical University, Carolo Wilhelmina, Brunswick, GFR.

21. Fuhrer, C. 1965. *Dtsch. Apoth-Ztg.*, 105:1150.

22. Ertel, K. D., B. Iyer, M. G. Williams and J. T. Carstensen. 1987. *Powder Techn.*, 52:101.

23. Khan, K. A. and C. T. Rhodes. 1975. *J. Pharm. Sci.*, 64:166.

24. Khan, K. A. and C. T. Rhodes. 1976. *J. Pharm. Sci.*, 65:1837.

25. Caramella, C., F. Ferrari, M. C. Bonferoni and M. Ronchi. 1990. *Drug Dev. Ind. Pharm.*, 116:2561.

26. Berry, H. and C. W. Ridout. 1950. *J. Pharm, Pharmacol.*, 2:619.

27. Kennon, L. and J. V. Swintosky. 1958. *J. Am. Pharm. Assoc., Sci. Ed.*, 47:397.

28. Couvreur, P. 1975. Thesis, Docteur en Sciences Pharmaceutiques, Univ. Catholique de Louvain, Belgium, p. 87.

5.17 PROBLEMS (CHAPTER 5)*

(1) You are an experienced development pharmacist, who is often called upon to make clinical batches for phase I studies of new compounds. To this end you have developed the following base formula, which you use when the drug content is below 10%.

Cornstarch	150 g
Lactose	1800 g
Cornstarch for paste	50 g

*Answers on pages 238, 239.

Crosspovidone	2%
Magnesium stearate	0.5%

(a) The base formula is made in the same manner as wet granulations are usually made. How would you add the crosspovidone and magnesium stearate:
  (1) Before the addition of cornstarch paste?
  (2) After the addition of cornstarch paste?
  (3) After the drying of the granulation of the other ingredients?
  (4) After drying and soft milling of the granulation of the other ingredients?

(b) You are asked to make a 10 mg tablet on a 1/4 " punch for phase I clinical trial. A 1/4 " punch makes tablets of weights of between 100 and 185 mg which have a thickness that is acceptable. You are given 300 g of drug substance.
  Give the composition for:
  (1) The formula of mg of each component per tablet.
  (2) The amounts and ingredients in the clinical batch, and the theoretical size of (number of tablets in) the batch. State the compression weight.

(c) You find that with the drug, the formulation doesn't flow quite as well as you want it to. What remedy would you try? (Note that you have already made the granulation, and cannot start from scratch.)

(d) Your remedy for improving the flow works, but you now find that the disintegration time has suffered and is too long. What remedy do you suggest?

(e) Your remedy works and you make the batch. Write the formula for ingredients per tablet and the formula used for the clinical batch (i.e., where the amount of drug = 300 g) (the batch record).

(f) What important machine instruction has been changed in your going from step (c) to (e)?

(2) You work for a manufacturer of excipients for the pharmaceutical industry. A new form of a food grade carbohydrate has been developed which shows great potential as a direct compression ingredient. You are asked to assemble physical data on the substance which supports this.

You determine that the true density is 1.25 g/cm³.

You make 0.5 gram tablets of this substance at a cross-sectional area of 1 cm² and at different compression pressures (expressed here in kg force/cm²) and measure their thickness. The following are the results.

2,000 kg force/cm²   thickness 9 mm
5,000 kg force/cm²   thickness 5 mm

(a) What is the yield value, ϕ? Show how you arrived at this and give units.

You next run hardness data as a function of applied pressure, with the results shown in Table 5.5.

(b) Draw the hardness/pressure profile, and explain the shape of the curve.
(c) Does the thickness at 7,000 kg force/cm² change your mind about your estimate of the yield value of the material?
(d) If the yield value of the most important competitor's product for your excipient is 1,000 (same units as above), would you consider the yield value of the carbohydrate a marketing advantage over the competitive product?
(e) In an experiment you obtain the following flow rate data into a 1/4″ die from mesh cuts of your material:

Size (μm)	100	200	300	400	500
grams/sec	1	4	6	9	10

If you think that the material should be capable of running on a high-speed machine making 30,000[13] 0.5 g[14] tablets per hour, using hoppers of a diameter of 5″, what is the particle size range you would recommend for the excipient? In your calculation, consider the feedframe to be 31.4 cm long and the diameter of the table to be 50 cm and assume there are sixty dies in the die table.

TABLE 5.5 Pressure/Hardness/Thickness Relations.

Pressure kg Force/cm²	Hardness kP	Thickness mm
2,000	4	9 mm
3,000	6	
4,000	8	
5,000	10	5 mm
7,000	11	6.8 mm

[13]Usually three hoppers each producing 30,000, so that a total of 90,000 are actually produced per hour.
[14]Tablet weight.

(3) A powder composition of drug and direct compression excipient is roller compacted, and then milled. Part of the material is compressed into a tablet, and part of it placed in a capsule. Both are subjected to dissolution testing and the results are listed below.

Capsule:

Time (min)	0	2	3	4	5	6	7
Amt. dissolved	0	20	60	80	90	95	97.5

Tablet:

Time (min)	0	6	7	8	9	10	11
Amt. dissolved	0	20	60	80	90	95	97.5

(a) Estimate the lag times. (You may do this graphically on a linear plot if you wish.)

(b) Although a tablet does not disintegrate into the particles from which it was made, the type of manufacture used here comes the closest, i.e., the particles into which the tablet disintegrates in the dissolution apparatus are fairly much the same size and shape as the ones from which the tablet was made.

Based on the above, estimate the wetting time (t_1) for the tablet and the penetration + disintegration time (t_2) for the tablet. Assume the wetting time to be the same for the tablet as for the capsule.[15]

---

[15]This is not strictly correct, because the area of wetting is more for the capsule than for the tablet.

CHAPTER 6

Granulation and Drying

The process of wet granulation has been referred to in the previous chapter, and the following will describe the process. The general purpose of wet granulation is (1) to enlarge the particle size, (2) to improve the particle shape (and make it fairly spherical), (3) to make the surface of the particles and the tablet hydrophilic (to promote wetting, and consequently disintegration and dissolution), and (4) to promote compressibility.

6.1 THE WET GRANULATION PROCESS

When wet granulating a dry solid, a binder is added to the mixture of the drug and (some of the) excipients. This "glues" particles together, so that they agglomerate into granules. These are quite spherical.

The most common binder is still cornstarch USP. Polyvinylpyrrolidone (PVP, polyplasdone) is frequently used, as are modified starches. Some of the latter are pregelatinized and will be referred to as such in the following. Some older binders are acacia and gelatin (and combinations of the two). Searches for new granulation agents are forever ongoing, e.g., such sources as sorghum starch have recently been investigated [1].

The manner in which a cornstarch paste is prepared is as follows. One part of cornstarch is added to one part of cold water, and a uniform suspension is produced by stirring. This is then added to nine parts of boiling water, and a translucent gel forms. This is a so-called 1:10 cornstarch paste. This is referred to as method A.

The order of addition can also be reversed, in which case more starch can be incorporated, but only an amount corresponding to 9% of the added water actually goes into the gel formation. This is referred to as method B.

That it is possible to produce two types of starch paste in this fashion is due to the temperature profile of the cornstarch. It is assumed below that cornstarch has a heat capacity of about 1.2 cal/g and water one of 1.0 cal/g. If nine parts of water at 100°C are added to one part of water and one part of starch at 25°C, then an intermediate temperature, t, is arrived at. The boiling water decreases in temperature by $(100 - t)$ degrees and the starch suspension increases in temperature by $(t - 25)$ degrees, so that t can be calculated by means of heat balance:

$$9 \times 1 \times (100 - t) = 1 \times 1 \times (t - 25) + 1 \times 1.2 \times (t - 25)$$

(6.1)

from which

$$955 = 11.2\, t \quad \text{or} \quad t = 85°C \tag{6.2}$$

The temperature profiles experienced by a 1:10 paste produced by methods A and B are shown in Figure 6.1, and it is obvious that the heat experience in method B is at lower temperatures than in A, so that less hydrolysis of the starch occurs.

As the starch paste is added to the mixture of drug and excipients [Figure 6.2(a)] it will start forming wet bridges between particles. In the beginning the wet paste is unevenly distributed [2,3] but will rapidly equilibrate [Figure 6.2(b)]. Once it is equilibrated, the agitation should be stopped, and this is a problem from a technological point of view. Let us first consider what will happen if it is not stopped at this point.

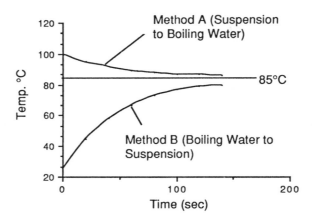

FIGURE 6.1. *Temperature of the starch particles when made by the two methods.*

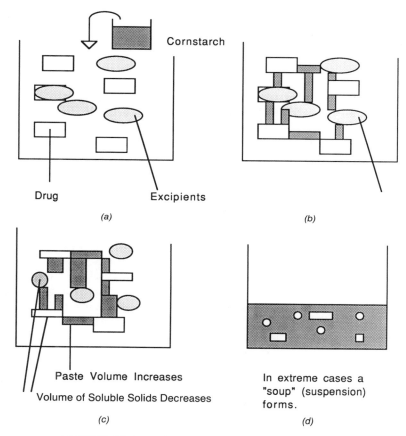

FIGURE 6.2. *Bond formation in the wet granulation mass.*

If some of the excipients, or the drug, are water soluble, then they will start to dissolve in the starch paste. This will make them smaller, and the "liquid phase" (i.e., the cornstarch paste) of larger volume. Hence the actual bond, when the granulation is dried, is largely a function of how long the granulation was kneaded. A higher temperature of paste increases hardness and disintegration time, due to the higher solids content of the binder bridges (more soluble excipient having had a chance to dissolve in the paste) [4].

In the limit the paste can "soup out," i.e., the liquid phase can become so large (and the solid phase conversely so small) that the solid phase no longer supports the liquid, and it simply turns into a suspension. The dissolution process is not nearly as rapid as in actual dissolution in water, because dissolution rates are retarded with increased viscosity of the medium. But souping out can occur in granulations if care is not taken.

The temperature of the addition of the starch is therefore important as well, because the higher the temperature, the higher the dissolution rate and the higher the solubility of the drug and excipients.

It is apparent from the above that granulations must be made with the greatest of care. In many cases one relies on operators to determine the "end point" of the granulations. This, however, is quite subjective, and automatic end point determination is often relied on nowadays. Here some torque measurements of the main drive are relied on, and discontinuities in the slope of power versus time curves, experimentally, fitted to the desired end point.

In development of a new drug product, it is common to rely on previous experience with drugs of a similar nature. Suppose a 250 mg tablet containing 10 mg of drug is the intended dosage form. Then, if it is desired to make 10,000 tablets, it would be necessary to use the quantities in Table 6.1.

In wet granulating, the "other excipients" in the table would include the wet granulating component of the formulation. Suppose the formula is planned as a lactose/cornstarch granulation. This type of granulation, for instance, could be known to work well for another similar product. Suppose, as well, that it is usually made in quantities of 1740 g (of granulation) and has the formula in the second column of Table 6.2. One now simply prorates by multiplying by 2476/1740, where 2476 is the amount of granulation calculated in Table 6.1.

Formulae are often arrived at in this fashion using a formula that is known to work to arrive at a new formula. If the new formula does not work, then revisions are made in it to make it work.

The master formula in Table 6.1 calls for the use of 2376 g of "other excipients." Since the first column in Table 6.2 contains 1740 g of excipient it is necessary to prorate the amounts of the latter by a factor of 2376/1740 as shown in the last column in Table 6.2.

TABLE 6.1 Basic Formula for a Tablet.

Ingredient	Amount per Tablet (mg)	Amount (g) per 10,000 Tablets
Drug	10 mg	100 g
Lubricant 1%	2.4 mg	24 g
Other Excipients	237.6 mg	2376 g
Total	250 mg	2500 g

TABLE 6.2 Formula for Excipients in Granulation of Cornstarch.

Excipient	Amount in Master Formula	Prorated Amount 2376/1740
Cornstarch	180 g	246 g
Lactose	1400 g	1912 g
Lactose for Preblend	115 g	157 g
Cornstarch for Paste	45 g	61 g
Total	1740 g	2376 g

There are three advantages in wet granulation procedures over direct compression:

(1) The wetting properties are better, particularly in the case of hydrophobic drug substances. The addition of the (usually) hydrophilic binder makes the surface of the hydrophobic drug more hydrophilic. This eases both disintegration and dissolution.

(2) The content uniformity is better. Ideally all the granules contain the same amount of drug substances, so that the only cause for lack of uniformity can come from the addition of the disintegrant and lubricant at the end. There are cases (soluble drugs) where the granule will act like a chromatogram, and the drug substance will wick to the surface as the granule dries [5]. In such cases there may still be content uniformity problems, but they are less than when pure powders are mixed. The distribution of active ingredient is a function of the consistency of the paste. The less viscous it is (i.e., the more dilute) the sharper the distribution curve is. As mentioned in another connection, the drug content is a function of the mesh cut, and sometimes increases with increasing particle size [6].

(3) The particle size and shape are optimized (as described earlier).

When pregelatinized starches are used, they are simply added to the powder mix, which is then granulated with water. Polyplasdone can be used the same way or it can be used by first making a solution and adding it, in the same manner a cornstarch paste is added. The mean particle size of the final granulation (all other factors being equal) is also a function of the amount of binder used [7].

Granulations are carried out in heavy duty mixing equipment known as kneaders. Typical are Hobart mixers (small), Sigma-type kneaders, and high-intensity mixers (V-blenders with intensifier bars, Lodige mixers with choppers, and present-day bowl mixers with impellers). Granulations can also be carried out in fluid bed driers (to be described below).

There is an ongoing research effort to improve the granulation procedures. (In fact, fluid bed granulation was such an improvement in the 1960s, and high-intensity bowl granulators in the 1970s.) Recently, continuous methods (continuous multi-purpose melt technology, CMT) [8] have been suggested as an improvement over present-day techniques. Here a granulating agent is melted and fluidized and pumped into a stream of the solid particles, and essentially enrobes them.

6.2 DRYING OF GRANULATIONS

After the end point is reached, the granulation is discharged from the kneader and must be dried. This type of drying takes place either in a traydryer (or truck-dryer) [7,9,10]. This consists of a series of large trays that are placed in a truck, which is then wheeled into an oven, where a flow of air across it will accomplish the drying of the granules (see Figure 6.3).

Less frequent is the use of vacuum dryers. In this case a so-called solids processer can be used. This is a large double-coned mixer, with ports for adding liquid, and for applying vacuum. The granulation is first formed and the vacuum then applied. In this way the transfer (traying) step is avoided.

It can also be carried out in fluid bed dryer [10], in which case it is referred to as a fluid bed granulator. These now also come with impellers.

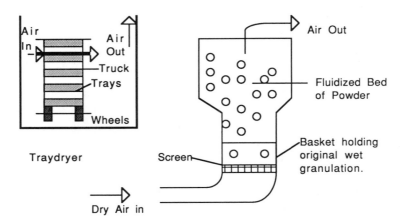

FIGURE 6.3. *Traydryer and fluid bed dryer.*

In recent years, the microwave dryer [11] has been successfully employed in granulation drying. The advantage here is the lower temperature needed. Water is usually removed by vacuum in such a case.

In all of the preceding cases there are several important drying end point considerations. Taking the example in Table 6.2, the 250 mg compression weight is predicated on the water content in the final formula being the same as it is in the raw materials listed. If a 1:10 paste is used, then 610 g of water would be present at the wet stage, and this is the amount that must be removed.

If more is removed, then the hydration water in lactose may be removed. One might say that that would be a simple matter to correct for, since one could simply adjust the fill weight. However, the lactose crystals "crumble" when they dehydrate, and the granule strength decreases. It is therefore crucial to monitor the correct end point of a granulation.

Example 6.1

The wet weight of a granulation made is shown in the second column with drug should be $2376 + 100 = 2476$ g, since it contains 100 g of drug and the wet granulation, assuming a 1:10 starch paste should contain 610 g of water as well so that the final wet weight should be 3086 g. In actuality (including losses) only 3000 g of wet mass was recovered. How much water (weight loss) should be removed in drying? What is the actual process loss?

Answer 6.1

The amount of water added is $10 \times 61 = 610$ g (since it is a 1:10 starch paste). The amount of water that must be removed is

$$610 \times 2400/2476 = 591 \text{ g}$$

The amount of dry solid is therefore $3000 - 591 = 2409$ grams.

If the drying process is monitored, then in pharmaceutical granulations the process is diffusional (constant rate drying [12]), i.e., if the amount of water per gram of dry solid,[16] Y is plotted logarithmically, versus time then

$$\ln [Y] = \ln [Y_o] - kt \qquad (6.3)$$

---

[16]"Dry" solid should be interpreted as solid that has the same water content as the "dry" raw materials used in the formula. Lactose is a hydrate, and the water of crystallization, in this context, is not counted as water, since it is part of the raw materials (and counts as such in the mg/tablet, at a tablet weight of 250 mg).

TABLE 6.3 Drying Data for a Granulation.

Time (hours)	Total Weight	Weight—2409 (grams water, Y)	ln [Y]
0	3000	591	6.382
3	2664	255	5.541
6	2519	110	4.700
9	2457	48	3.871
12	2430	21	3.045
15	2417.8	8.8	2.175
18	2412.8	3.8	1.335
21	2410.7	1.7	0.531
24	2409.7	0.7	−0.357
48	2400*		
60	2390*		
96	2380*		

*These samples are excessively dried.

Example 6.2

The granulation just described is dried in a traydryer at 50°C. The characteristics in Table 6.3 result.

What is the recommended maximum drying time, and how do the data plot rationally?

Answer 6.2

It is obvious from the table (and from Figure 6.4), that somewhere between 24 and 48 hours the weight will go below 2409 (which is the weight

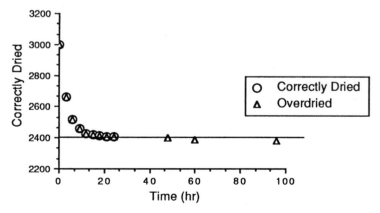

FIGURE 6.4. Data from Figure 6.3 plotted on linear (Cartesian) coordinates.

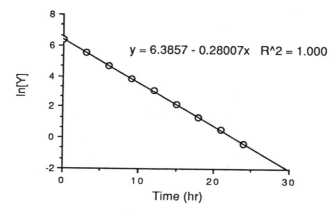

FIGURE 6.5. *Data from the falling rate period plotted according to Equation (6.3).*

of the dry materials), and hence 24 hours would be the maximum (and recommended) drying time.

In the table, Y has been calculated by subtracting 2409 from the weight figures. The logarithm has been taken and is plotted in Figure 6.5. Obviously, Equation (6.3) is obeyed.

In fluid bed drying, the dry inlet air has a higher temperature than the air in the expansion chamber, so that the exit air will maintain a lower temperature during the drying. The moment the granulation is dry, the exit air temperature will increase (because water is no longer being evaporated, and hence there is no caloric requirement on the stream anymore). This can be used to shut off the dryer automatically, so that the type of overdrying in Table 6.3 (last three lines) and Figure 6.4 does not occur.

It should be pointed out that just as granules leave a dryer, the larger particles have a higher moisture content than the smaller particles. In most cases the moisture will equilibrate between the various mesh cuts [13,14].

6.3 REFERENCES

1. Garr, J. S. M. and A. B. Bangudu. 1991. *Drug Dev. Ind. Pharm.*, 17:2.
2. Zoglio, M. A., W. H. Streng and J. Carstensen. 1975. *J. Pharm. Sci.*, 64:1869.
3. Zoglio, M. A., H. E. Huber, G. Koehne, P. L. Chan and J. T. Carstensen. 1976. *J. Pharm. Sci.*, 65:12054.
4. Pilpel, N. and S. Esezobo. 1977. *J. Pharm. Pharmacol.*, 29:389.
5. Rubenstein, M. H. and K. Ridgeway. 1974. *J. Pharm. Pharmacol.*, 26:24P.
6. Selkirk, A. B. 1976. *J. Pharm. Pharmacol.*, 28:512.
7. Carstensen, J. T., F. Puisieux, A. Mehta and M. A. Zoglio. 1978. *Int. J. Pharm.*, 1:65.

8. Appelgren, C. and C. Eskilson. 1990. *Drug Dev. Ind. Pharm.*, 16:2345.

9. Samaha, N. W., N. A. ElGindy and ElMaradny. 1986. *Pharm. Ind.*, 48:193.

10. Travers, D. N. 1975. *J. Pharm. Pharmacol*, 27:516.

11. VanScoik, K., M. A. Zoglio and J. T. Carstensen. 1991. "Drying and Driers," In *Encyclopedia of Pharmaceutical Technology*, J. Swarbrick and J. C. Boylan, eds., New York, NY: Marcel Dekker, p. 494.

12. VanScoik, K., M. A. Zoglio and J. T. Carstensen. 1991. "Drying and Driers," In *Encyclopedia of Pharmaceutical Technology*, J. Swarbrick and J. C. Boylan, eds., New York, NY: Marcel Dekker, pp. 510–513.

13. Carstensen, J. T. and M. A. Zoglio. 1979. "Drying," *Am. Pharm. Assoc. Meeting, Kansas City, MO, Nov. 1979, Abstracts*, p. 10.

14. Pitkin, C. and J. T. Carstensen. 1973. *J. Pharm. Sci.*, 62:1215.

6.4 PROBLEMS (CHAPTER 6)*

(1) A granulation is made with the following overall formula:

Cornstarch (containing 7% moisture)	15%
Microcrystalline cellulose (with 5% moisture)	20%
Lactose (4% moisture)	35%
Drug (anhydrous)	30%

All percentages are g of water per 100 g of solid "as-is." What should the moisture specification be for the final granulation after drying?

(2) Forty grams of water is added to 600 g of dry solid for granulation purposes and then dried. After 8 hours the weight is 620 g. What is the drying rate constant? Assume the weight levels out at 600 g.

CHAPTER 7

Stability of Solid Dosage Forms

The stability of solid dosage forms will be shortly overviewed here. For a deeper insight into this, other texts are recommended [1]. In solutions, most decompositions are hydrolyses. In such a case, the decomposition is first order [1–3]:

$$dC/dt = -kC \qquad (7.1)$$

It has been mentioned that in solutions there is not the content uniformity problem that is encountered in solids, and it is often possible to determine that a solution that has decomposed, e.g., to an extent of 7% is, indeed, first order. In the case of solid dosage forms, the content uniformity would prevent such conclusions. Nevertheless, the stability of a substance in solution is tied into what it is in the solid dosage form, since this latter is never a completely anhydrous entity.

7.1 STABILITY OF SOLID IN THE PRESENCE OF MOISTURE

One of the advantages of solid dosage forms vis-a-vis liquid dosage forms is that they, in general, are more stable. However, it is primarily moisture in the dosage form that causes its instability, and hence there is a link between solution and solid state stability.

It is known that drugs in solution usually decompose by hydrolysis, e.g., aspirin would decompose by the reaction

$$C_6H_4(OOCCH_3)COOH + H_2O \rightarrow C_6H_4(OH)COOH + CH_3COOH$$

$$(7.2)$$

The decomposition rate is proportional to both the concentration of aspirin and of water [4]. If the beginning concentration, $[A]$, of aspirin were 0.1 molar, then it would be zero molar at the "completion" of the reaction. Water is, however, 1000/18 molar $= 55.6$ molar. At the end of the reaction it would be 55.5 molar, i.e., hardly have changed at all. The rate equation would hence be

$$dC/dt = -k_2[A][H_2O] = k_1[A] \tag{7.3}$$

where

$$k_1 = k_2[H_2O] \tag{7.4}$$

is called the pseudo–first order rate constant.

It is obvious from what has been described about the manufacture of solid dosage forms that the dosage forms always contain some water. This water acts as a "solution medium," and all the decomposition (usually) takes place in this aqueous layer (Figure 7.1). It is assumed that the concentration of drug in the aqueous layer is the saturation concentration (solubility, S). It is further assumed that each time a molecule decomposes in the liquid layer, it is replaced by one that dissolves from the solid phase, so that the aqueous layer is *always* saturated in drug. Under these conditions the rate equation in the aqueous layer becomes:

$$dC/dt = -k_1 S \tag{7.5}$$

i.e., the rate is a constant. If there is an amount (volume), V (g or cm^3) of water in the dosage form, then the amount (M gram) of drug lost (dM) is obtained by multiplying the volume by the loss concentration ($-dC$), i.e.

$$dM/dt = [-dC/dt]V = k_1 SV = k_o \tag{7.6}$$

Hence, the amount of drug lost per time unit is a constant, so the reaction will appear as if it were zero order. This is called pseudo–zero order, and k_o is called the pseudo–zero order rate constant. Equation (7.6) may be integrated:

$$M = M_o - (k_1 VS)t = M_o - k_o t \tag{7.7}$$

This means that the more water there is in a dosage form, the more unstable it is going to be.

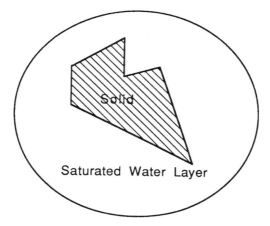

FIGURE 7.1. *Schematic of decomposition in a solid dosage form containing available moisture.*

Example 7.1

A vitamin A tablet loses 20% of its potency after three years on the shelf at room temperature. The tablets contain 1% moisture. Another batch of tablets contains 2% moisture. How much will they lose?

Answer 7.1

Since the percent moisture is twice as high in the second batch they will lose potency twice as fast, and will lose 40% after three years.

It is noted, therefore, that the rate constant of the decomposition is given by:

$$k_1 SV = k_o \qquad (7.8)$$

Hence, if the apparent rate constant is plotted versus the moisture content, then a straight line through the origin should result. Most often, however, this is not quite the case. There is a lower limit, below which the moisture is "bound," and there is, below this limit, no aqueous layer [5], i.e., the product is quite stable below this limit:

$$k_o = \beta + k_1 SV \qquad (7.9)$$

where β is quite low. This is shown in Figures 7.2 and 7.3.

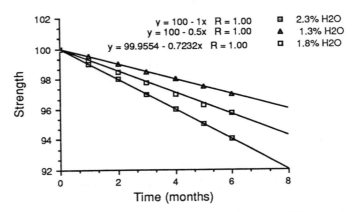

FIGURE 7.2. *Pseudo–zero order reaction in the solid state at different moisture contents.*

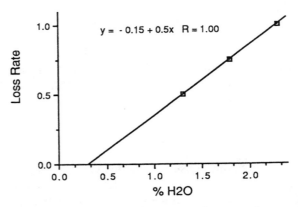

FIGURE 7.3. *Effect of moisture content on pseudo–zero order rate constant.*

108

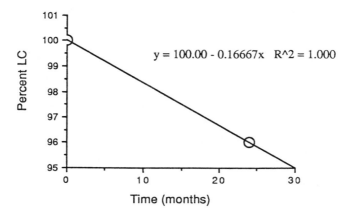

FIGURE 7.4. *Two-point stability example. Note that the abscissa is in units of months. (The text uses years as a unit.)*

7.2 STATISTICS OF THE STRAIGHT LINE (LINEAR REGRESSION)

To investigate the stability of a drug substance it is necessary to have at least two points: an initial assay and an assay after a given storage period, t (e.g., 24 months). This is depicted in Figure 7.4. It is obvious that it is not possible to state what the order of the reaction is. If it were, e.g., zero order (noting from Figure 7.4 that 4% is lost in two years), then the rate constant would be 2% per year. This would extrapolate to a strength of 94.00% after three years. If it were first order, however, then:

$$\ln (0.96) = -0.0408 = k \times 2 \quad \text{or} \quad k = 0.0204 \text{ years} \quad (7.10)$$

This would extrapolate to

$$\ln (x) = -0.0204 \times 3 - 0.0608, \text{ i.e., } x = 0.941 = 94.10\% \quad (7.11)$$

Although the differences are not great in this case, the fact is that a different number is arrived at, so that by a two-point method, extrapolations become, from the perspective of the model, unsound.

Furthermore, the precision becomes highly important. If the standard deviation of the assay is 0.02 (i.e., 2%), then the variance on the difference $(100 - 96 = 4\%)$ becomes:

$$s^2 = 0.02^2 + 0.02^2 = 0.0008 \quad (7.12)$$

so that the standard deviation on the difference is $\sqrt{0.0008} =$ ca. 0.03 (or 3%). The standard deviation of the rate constant would be about half that, and that of the extrapolated strength at 3 years would be 1.5 times 3%, i.e., about 5%. These are data used to exemplify the problem, and the first point to make is that, for order of reaction and statistical evaluation, at least three points are needed.

The point is that only one line can be fitted through two points, hence two points give no information about precision. One says that the degrees of freedom are $N - 2$ in the case of a line (just like they are $N - 1$ in the case of an average).

Since there is only one line, it is possible to give one (and only one) equation describing the line:

$$y = \text{intercept} + (\text{slope} \times x) = a + bx \qquad (7.13)$$

where, as indicated, a is y-intercept and b is slope. This latter is obtained from the two points (x_1, y_1) and (x_2, y_2) as:

$$b = (y_1 - y_2)/(x_1 - x_2) \qquad (7.14)$$

and the equation is given by:

$$y - y_1 = b(x - x_1) \qquad (7.15)$$

i.e., the intercept is:

$$y_1 - bx_1 \qquad (7.16)$$

If more points are available, then the situation in Figure 7.5 results. This is an example, and the precision of the data is unrealistically high. The equation for the line can be obtained from any two points (in this highly precise example) by the use of Equations (7.14) to (7.16).

A more realistic example is shown in Figure 7.6. For the sake of example these data are very imprecise.

Many investigators have a tendency to want to simply connect the points by line segments, as is done, e.g., in a patient's temperature chart (Figure 7.7).

But recall that the points scatter because of assay, because of sample, and because of storage variation, not because of the order of the reaction or the general stability trend. What must be done is to draw a line through the points in the best manner possible. It would seem rational to draw the line so that as many points were above as below, but even that can be done in many manners. Suppose, as shown in Figure 7.8, that two persons draw

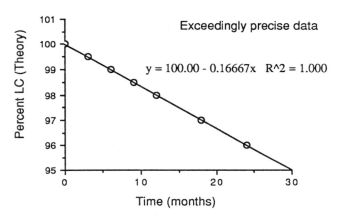

FIGURE 7.5. *Example of highly precise data of a linear nature.*

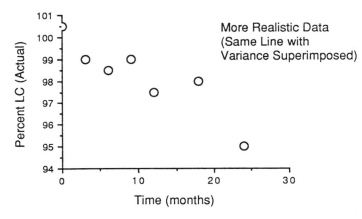

FIGURE 7.6. *Example of imprecise data of a linear nature. The data are actually the data in Figure 7.5 with a variance imposed on them.*

111

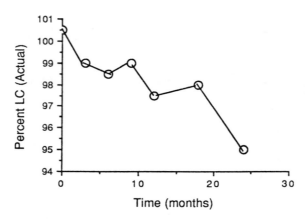

FIGURE 7.7. *Improper treatment of data in Figure 7.6.*

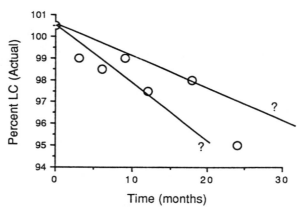

FIGURE 7.8. *Two "eyeballed" lines drawn through data from Figure 7.6. Which is the "better" line?*

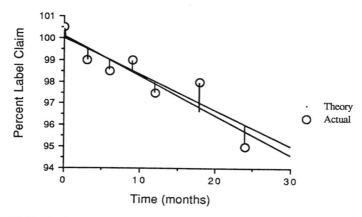

FIGURE 7.9. *The least squares fit line from Figure 7.8. Shown with the theoretical line (which is ordinarily not known) and the line that is estimated from the experimental data.*

each what they think is a best line, simply by eye. The question then is, which is the best line?

In order to arbitrate an argument as to which line is the best it is (as in all selection processes) necessary to have a rule or a set of rules. By definition the "best" line is defined as follows. If the distances from the points to the line are drawn (see Figure 7.9) and denoted Δ, then the one and only line that has the smallest sum of Δ^2 is denoted the least squares fit line, and is usually considered the best choice for a line through the points given.[17]

The formulae for slope and intercept are as follows:

$$\text{Slope} = a = [\Sigma(xy) - (\Sigma x \Sigma y/N)]/[\Sigma x^2 - (\{\Sigma x\}^2/N)] \quad (7.17)$$

$$\text{Intercept} = b = (\Sigma y - a\Sigma x)/N \quad (7.18)$$

This will be exemplified with the simple three-point case listed in Table 7.1. It is then seen that the slope has the value:

$$a = [288 - \{(3 \times 292.9)/3\}]/[5 - (3^2/3)] = -4.9/2 = -2.45 \quad (7.19)$$

---

[17]This is somewhat akin to accepting the average to be the best representative of a set of numbers. The average has, for the set, the least sum of squares of any number.

TABLE 7.1 Three-Point Stability Data Used to Exemplify Equations (7.17) and (7.18).

Time (x)	Strength (y)	x^2	xy	y^2
0	100	0	0	10,000
1	97.8	1	97.8	9,564.84
2	95.1	4	190.2	9,044.01
$\Sigma = 3$	292.9	5	288	28,608.85

The intercept is given by:

$$b = [292.9 - (-2.45 \times 3)]/3$$

$$= (292.9 + 7.35)/3 = 300.4/3 = 100.08 \qquad (7.20)$$

The strength after three years can be calculated to be

$$y_{36}^{\wedge} = 100.08 - (2.45 \times 3) = 100.08 - 7.35 = 92.73 = 92.7$$

$$(7.21)$$

This is an estimate of the population average at the three-year point, and half of the time it will be too high, half of the time too low. The experimental points are denoted y, and the points on the least squares fit line (at any x) are denoted $y^{\wedge}$.

A property that is of importance is the sum of squares, $\Sigma\Delta^2$. This is calculated in Table 7.2, where the point on the line, $y^{\wedge}$, is calculated for each of the experimental x-values.

TABLE 7.2 Example of Least Squares Fit Calculations.

Time (yr)	y	$y^{\wedge}$	Δ	Δ^2
0	100	100.08	-0.08	0.0064
1	97.8	97.633	0.166	0.0276
2	95.1	95.183	-0.083	0.0069
Total				0.0409

The sum of the deviations squared is

$$\Sigma(y - y^\wedge)^2 = 0.0409 \qquad (7.22)$$

The equivalent of a variance is denoted s_{yx}^2, and is the above number divided by the degrees of freedom, i.e.

$$s_{yx}^2 = [\Sigma(y - y^\wedge)^2]/(N - 2) = 0.0409/1 = 0.0490 \qquad (7.23)$$

so that

$$s_{yx} = [0.0490]^{1/2} = 0.22 \qquad (7.24)$$

A quantity frequently used is the correlation coefficient, R, which is given by:

$$R^2 = [\Sigma(xy) - (\Sigma x \Sigma y/N)]^2/\{[\Sigma x^2 - (\{\Sigma x\}^2/N)][\Sigma y^2 - (\{\Sigma y\}^2/N)]\} \qquad (7.25)$$

The closer R is to either plus or minus one, the better the correlation. The significance of the correlation is a function of the number of points that have been used, a point that will not be belabored here.

The above is shown as an example. Nowadays the values of a, b, and R can be gotten from most calculators, and good Stat programs exist for virtually all types of computers. (The system is quite easy to program, in any event [6].)

7.3 CONFIDENCE LIMITS ABOUT EXTRAPOLATED POINTS

Confidence limits involve questions such as the following: If one states that an assay is, say 95.2%, then how "correct" is this? Obviously there are several sources of error, so that one usually attaches limits on the number, e.g., 95.2% ± 0.5%. Such limits are usually 95% confidence limits, which means that one is 95% sure that the average is to be found in the interval 94.7–95.7% [7–10].

For numbers the confidence limit is the average ±

$$t_{n-1,\alpha}s(1/n)^{1/2} \qquad (7.26)$$

TABLE 7.3 Two-Sided Student t-Values at the 95% and 90% Confidence Level* with ν Degrees of Freedom.

Degrees of Freedom	$t_{n-1,\alpha}$ — 95% One-Sided 90% Two-Sided	$t_{n-1,\alpha}$ — 95% Two-Sided
1	6.31	12.71
2	2.92	4.30
3	2.35	3.18
4	2.13	2.77
5	2.02	2.57
6	1.94	2.45
7	1.90	2.37
8	1.86	2.31
10	1.81	2.23
16	1.75	2.12
∞	1.65	1.96

*It is to be noted that two-sided at 90% is equivalent to one-sided at 95% confidence.

where s is the standard deviation and t is the Student t-value for the given number of degrees of freedom. A compilation of such values is shown in Table 7.3.

For an extrapolated value in a linear regression, the expression for the 90% confidence limit is:

$$\gamma = t_{(0.90,N-2)}s_{yx}[(1/N) + \{(x - x_{avg})^2/(\Sigma(x - x_{avg})^2\}]^{1/2} \quad (7.27)$$

i.e., there is a 90% probability that the population mean (in a manner of speaking, "the true value") lies in the interval

$$y^\Delta \pm \gamma \quad (7.28)$$

Since this is symmetric, there is a 5% chance the true value is below $y^\Delta - \gamma$ and a 5% chance the true value is above $y^\Delta + \gamma$. Since we are not interested in the latter (it is drop in potency which concerns us), the expression in Equation (7.27) is also the expression for the lower 95% confidence limit that the assay at the extrapolated time will be above

$$y^\Delta - \gamma \quad (7.29)$$

This is a one-sided test (above, not in-between) which is the reason for using t for 90% two-sided (the same as 95% one-sided).

In the example in Table 7.2, we can now determine the 90% confidence bound about $y^\wedge(3)$ to be:

$$6.3 \times 0.22 \times (\sqrt{[(1/3) + \{(3 - 1)^2/2\}]} = 1.386 \times \sqrt{2.3} = 2.1$$

(7.30)

so that

$$y^\wedge(36) = 92.7 \pm 2.1 > 90\% \text{ of label claim} \qquad (7.31)$$

The correlation coefficient, R, is given by Equation (7.25), so

$$R^2 = [\Sigma(xy) - (\Sigma x \Sigma y/N)]^2/\{[\Sigma x^2 - (\{\Sigma x\}^2/N)] [\Sigma y^2 - (\{\Sigma y\}^2/N)]$$

$$= [288 - (3 \times 292.9/3)]^2/[5 - (3^2/3)][28{,}608.85 - (292.92^2/3)]$$

$$= 0.996 \qquad (7.32)$$

Suppose, as in Example 7.1, there are good data, but a small N, and a long extrapolation. In this case (Figure 7.10) the confidence band becomes broad, because N is small ($1/N$ is large) and the term $(x_{avg} - x_{extrapolated})^2$ becomes large.

The situation improves with a small s, a small N, and short extrapolation, because now the term $(x_{avg} - x_{extrapolated})^2$ becomes smaller (Figure 7.11).

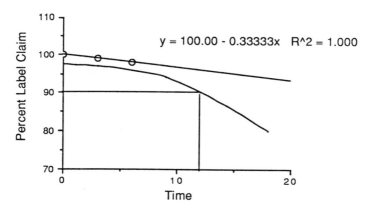

FIGURE 7.10. *Small N, good data, long extrapolation.*

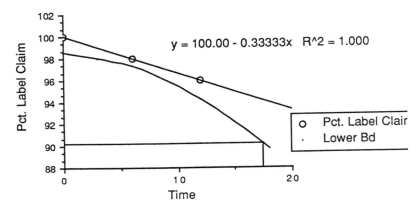

FIGURE 7.11. *Small s_{yx}, small N, short extrapolation.*

With a small s_{yx}, a larger N, and a short extrapolation, the confidence band gets even narrower (Figure 7.12).

Often, the data are quite scattered (i.e., s_{yx} is large). Such an example is shown in Figure 7.13.

The actual method used in the FDA Stability Guideline of 1987 is one where the least squares fit line is drawn for the N data points, the "variance," s_{yx} is then calculated and the value:

$$x - t_{0.95,N-2}s_{yx}[(1/N) + \{(x - x_{avg})/\Sigma(x - x_{avg})\}]^{1/2} \qquad (7.33)$$

is calculated for a series of points, and is called the lower confidence bound.

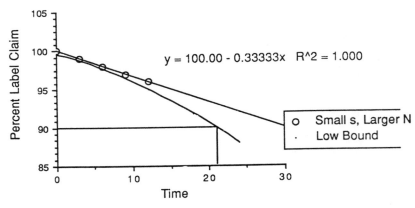

FIGURE 7.12. *Small s, larger N, short extrapolation.*

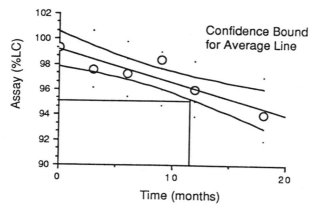

FIGURE 7.13. *Large s, intermediate N, short extrapolation.*

The point where this line cuts the line $y = 90\% \, LC$ is the expiration period (Figure 7.14) [8,9].

7.4 EXPIRATION DATING

It would be nice if all products were 100% stable, but all drug substances have the potential for loss in strength. The FDA guidelines essentially require that a manufacturer state on the label what the drug content of the tablet is (what its label claim, LC, is). If this were true initially, then as the dosage form was stored it would degrade, and it would no longer meet the

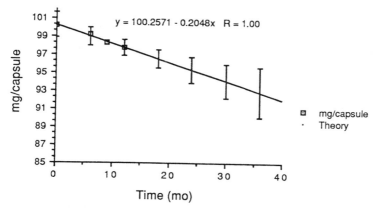

FIGURE 7.14. *Expiration period calculation.*

requirement. Secondly, it is impossible (unlike in the case of liquids) to make a batch of tablets where each tablet contains exactly the same amount. This is one of the reasons that there are specification limits set in the USP for all products. These are usually 90–110% of label claim (LC).

The loss rate of the product in Figure 7.15 is 0.2 mg/month. First of all one should note that if the product contained 10 mg of drug, then this would amount to 2% per month, but if the product contained 100 mg of drug, then it would represent 0.2% per month. Hence, in zero and pseudo–zero order decompositions it is important to realize the effect of the strength. There are many products on the market that exhibit good stability in the higher dosage forms, but marginal stability in the lower dosage forms.

It would be tempting to calculate the expiration period of, e.g., the 100 mg product by saying that since it loses 0.2% per month, it will take fifty months to lose 10%, and if the specification limits are 90–110%, then that would represent the time when the average potency would drop to the lower specification limit.

The manufacturer must specify an expiration date. This is calculated by determining the stability profile of the drug, and is exemplified below.

Example 7.2

A particular formulation of tetracycline capsules exhibits the stability shown in Table 7.4.

How much strength would remain after three years?

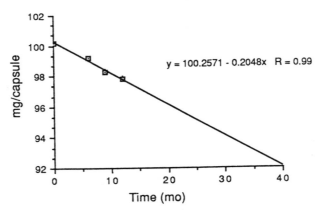

FIGURE 7.15. Typical zero order decomposition.

TABLE 7.4 Example of Stability of a Solid Dosage Form.

Time (months)	Strength	Strength (mg/capsule)
0	100	100.2
6	99	99.2
9	98.5	98.3
12	98	97.8

Answer 7.2

It is seen that in the first case (second column) the loss rate is exactly 2 mg/capsule per year, so that exactly 6 mg would be lost after three years of storage. The 94% remaining is well above the lower specification limit (90% LC), so that if these data were realistic, three years' expiration would be granted.

The last column is a much more realistic situation. The data are assumed to be linear, and are treated by least squares fitting. This gives the equation (Figure 7.15):

$$M = 100.26 - 0.205x \qquad (7.34)$$

hence, the average amount left after three years at room temperature is

$$M(36 \text{ months}) = 92.9 \qquad (7.35)$$

This is, however, the average amount, i.e, if the experiment were repeated 100 times, then the average would be less half of the time.

It is desired to predict expiration with a certainty of 95%, i.e., to do it in such a fashion that the true average is above the predicted potency 95 cases out of 100. As seen above it is possible to calculate the so-called 95% confidence limits about this extrapolated number. In this case, the prediction would be within the limits 95 times out of 100. These limits are 1.5,

$$M(36 \text{ months}) = 92.9 \pm 1.5 \qquad (7.36)$$

If the lower figure is higher than 90% LC (or the lower specification limit), then the product has an expiration date of three years.

7.5 SLOPE METHOD FOR DETERMINING EXPIRATION DATES

As mentioned, the guidelines, aside from requiring that expiration dates be placed on labels, also require that the company be 95% certain that the average of the drug content of each lot marketed contains above 90% label claim. The procedures would guarantee this 95% of the time. If only the least squares fit line had been used, then this could be guaranteed only 50% of the time.

The easiest way to explain the difference between simple loss rate calculations and the actual expiration period calculation is as follows.

Suppose a batch of a product were tested,[18] and the following data found:

Initial assay – 100% LC
Twelve months at room temperature – 98% LC

Provided (and we shall assume so in theory) that the assay was completely accurate and precise, we might then state that the yearly loss rate was 2% per year, so that after three years there would be 94% LC left.

However if two other batches B and C were tested, then the results might have been as shown in Table 7.5.

It can be seen from statistical tables that 68% of all (normally distributed) data are between the average ± one standard deviation. That means that 32% are outside, and for symmetry reasons, 16% of the data points are below the average minus one standard deviation and 68 + 16 = 84% of the numbers are below the average plus one standard deviation.

Similarly, 95% of all (normally distributed) data are between the average ± two standard deviations. That means that 5% are outside, and for symmetry reasons, 2.5% of the data points are below the average minus two standard deviations and 95 + 2.5 = 97.5% of the numbers are below the average plus two standard deviations.

TABLE 7.5 Decomposition of Three Batches of a Product.

	A	B	C
Initial assay	100	101	99
Assay after 12 months	98	98.5	97.5
Loss rates % per year	2	2.5	1.5

[18]Many more than two points are used in reality; the two points are used here for the sake of simplicity.

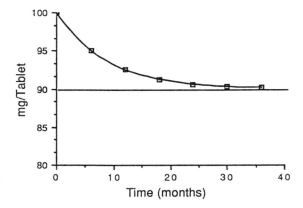

FIGURE 7.16. *Decomposition in the presence of limited amounts of water.*

If, in the previous data, the average initial assay is 100% LC with a standard deviation of 1%, then we may be at least 97.5% sure (two standard deviations) that the initial assay will be above $100 - 2 = 98\%$.

If the average rate constant is 2% per year with a standard deviation of 0.5% per year, we may be at least 97.5% sure (two standard deviations) that it is less than $2 + (2 \times 0.5) = 3\%$ per year.

If the initial assay was 98% and the loss rate was 3% per year, then the lower label claim, 90% LC, would have been reached in $8/3 = 2.3$ years, and this would (in this calculation mode) be the allowable expiration period.

The method described is simplified, but shows the fallacy of the simple (and incorrect) view that all that has to be done is draw a line through the stability points, and where this line cuts 90% LC is where the shelf life is.

Typically the expiration period is three years, sometimes, in the case of very stable drugs, it is four years.

In the case where there is only a very limited amount of moisture present, the decomposition cannot exceed the number of moles of moisture present, and the decomposition will have the profile shown in Figure 7.16.

7.6 ACCELERATED TESTING

The one accelerated test employed in the guidelines is a storage of the drug product in its container and package at 75% RH at 40°C (the Joel Davis Test). If the product holds up for three months under these conditions (chemical stability, dissolution, physical characteristics), then in an

ANDA, the generic company will be given a two-year expiration date, but must follow up with real time data to substantiate the dating. The method is, however, also used by ethical companies in the development of new drug entities. If the product does not pass the Joel Davis test, then conventional stability testing at room temperature for prolonged periods (eighteen months) must accompany the NDA or the ANDA to satisfy the stability requirements of the submission.

For formula evaluation, or where formula changes are made, accelerated testing at elevated temperatures is often carried out. Marketed containers are usually polyethylene, and since the dosage form will dry out if the bottle is simply placed in a high degree oven,[19] the dosage form in the (anticipated) marketed container is usually placed in a larger glass container (of volume V_{large}). The assembly is then placed at the high temperature station. The largest amount of moisture (g) that can be lost from the dosage form in this case would be:

$$18\,n = 18\,PV_{large}/RT \tag{7.37}$$

In such a case, it is often possible to extrapolate [10] the findings from the high-temperature data to room-temperature data. The equation used for this is the Arrhenius equation:

$$\ln[k] = \ln[Z] - (E/R)(1000/T) \tag{7.38}$$

where k is rate constant, Z is a pre-exponential factor (the collision factor), E is activation energy in kcal/deg, R is the gas constant in cal/deg/mole, and T is the absolute temperature. The use of this is exemplified in Example 7.3, below.

Example 7.3

Suppose a product was placed at different temperatures and the results shown in Table 7.6[20] were obtained.

TABLE 7.6 Example of Accelerated Data.

Storage Temperature	Assay Months	(% Label Claim)
55°C	1	85
45°C	1	95

[19]It shall be seen in a later chapter that only glass is actually completely moisture-impermeable.
[20]Many more than two points are used in reality. The two points are used here for sake of simplicity.

TABLE 7.7 Arrhenius Calculations of Data from Table 7.5.

Temperature °C	Temperature K	1000/T K^{-1}	k mo^{-1}	ln [k]
55	328	3.049	0.1625	−1.817
45	318	3.145	0.0513	−2.970
25	298	3.356	?	?

Estimate the rate constant at 25°C (k_{25}). Assume first order.

Answer 7.3

First order requires that

$$\ln [C/C_o] = -kt \text{ or } k = -(1/t) \ln [C/C_o] \qquad (7.39)$$

where C is drug content at time t and C_o is initial drug content. (Hence, e.g., for 85% retained, $[C/C_o]$ is equal to 0.85.)

The rate constants and their logarithms are:

55°C:

$$k = -\ln [0.85] = 0.1625 \qquad (7.40)$$

$$\ln [k_{55}] = -1.817 \qquad (7.41)$$

45°C:

$$k = -\ln [0.95] = 0.0513 \qquad (7.42)$$

$$\ln k = -2.970 \qquad (7.43)$$

Convert the temperatures to absolute temperatures by adding 273 (e.g., 55°C = 55 + 273 = 328 K), and take the reciprocals of this. This gives the set of data shown in Table 7.7. (The log of the rate constants is also shown in this table.)

ln [k] is plotted versus 1000/T. The equation is (0 df)

$$\ln [k] = 34.803 - 12.01(1000/T) \qquad (7.44)$$

The activation energy is given by:

$$-E/R = -12.01, \text{ so } E = 1.99 \times 12.01 = 24 \text{ kcal/mole} \qquad (7.45)$$

To find the room temperature constant from this, the value $1000/T = 3.356$ is inserted in Equation (7.44):

$$\ln [k_{2s}] = 34.803 - (12.01 \times 3.356)$$

$$= 34.803 - 40.339 = -5.536 \qquad (7.46)$$

so that

$$k = \exp(-5.536) = 0.004 \text{ mo}^{-1} \qquad (7.47)$$

After thirty-six months at 25°C, the estimated, extrapolated amount retained is given by:

$$\ln [C/C_o] = -0.004 \times 36 = -0.144 \qquad (7.48)$$

or

$$C/C_o = 0.866 = 86.6\% \qquad (7.49)$$

There are usually more points than two. An example of this is shown in Figure 7.17.

Again, the rate constants are obtained from the slopes of the lines, their logarithms are taken and plotted versus $1000/T$. This is shown in Figure 7.18.

It is noted that one problem with this is the calculation of the confidence limits [11–14] $N = 3$, so there is only one degree of freedom, and t (Table 7.3) becomes 12.7! Hence the confidence interval at the extrapolated value at 25°C would become exceedingly large, and calculating the expiration period by the slope method would probably result in the strength being somewhere between 0 and 100%.

But the fact remains that there are 18 points plus initial assays, so there should actually be $18 - 2 = 16$ degrees of freedom, so that the t-value should equal 1.75, not 12.7. One way to take advantage of the many points [15–17] is to note that (since $-\ln [C/C_o] = \ln [C_o/C]$):

$$k = (1/t) \ln [C_o/C] \qquad (7.50)$$

and that therefore the Arrhenius equation can be written:

$$\ln [k] = \ln \{(1/t) \ln [C_o/C]\} = (E/R)(1000/T) + \ln Z \quad (7.51)$$

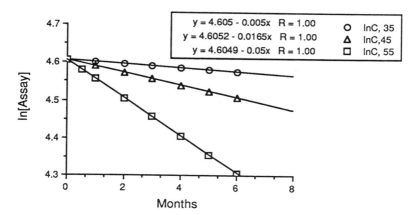

FIGURE 7.17. *Multipoint accelerated data study.*

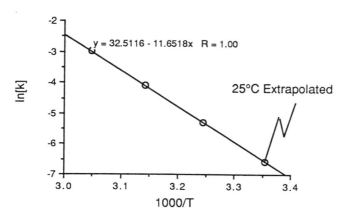

FIGURE 7.18. *Data from Figure 7.17 treated by Arrhenius treatment.*

so that regressing ln $\{(1/t)\ \ln\ [C_o/C]\}$ versus $1000/T$ will give a slope of E/R and an intercept of ln Z. Extrapolations are much more meaningful (i.e., the confidence limits of percent retained after thirty-six months are much narrower) when the plotting is carried out in this manner, because the degrees of freedom and N will both be larger, and hence t will be smaller.

7.7 REFERENCES

1. Carstensen, J. T. 1989. *Drug Stability*. New York, NY: Marcel Dekker.
2. Nikfar, F., S. J. Forbes, K. G. Mooney and J. T. Carstensen. 1990. *Pharm. Res.*, 7, S.182.
3. Nikfar, F., S. Ku, K. G. Mooney and J. T. Carstensen. 1990. *Pharm. Res.*, 7, S.127.
4. Carstensen, J. T. and F. Attarchi. 1988. *J. Pharm. Sci.*, 77:318.
5. Gerhardt, A. 1990. Ph.D. thesis, University of Wisconsin, Madison, WI 53706.
6. Carstensen, J. T. 1990. *Drug Stability*. New York, NY: Marcel Dekker.
7. Carstensen, J. T. 1977. *Pharmaceutics of Solids and Solid Dosage Forms*. New York, NY: Wiley, p. 8.
8. Carstensen, J. T. and E. Nelson. 1976. *J. Pharm. Sci.*, 65:311.
9. Langenbucher, F. 1990. *Drug. Dev. Ind. Pharm.*, 17:165.
10. Carstensen, J. T., F. Nikfar, T. Morris and A. Gerhardt. 1990. *Drug Dev. Ind. Pharm.*, 16:2267.
11. Carstensen, J. T. and K. Su. 1972. *J. Pharm. Sci.*, 61:223.
12. King, S.-Y. P., M.-S. Kung and H.-L. Fung. 1984. *J. Pharm. Sci.*, 73:657.
13. Carstensen, J. T. 1978. "How Long and at What Risk?" paper presented at the *17th Ann. Conf. Pharm. Analysis, University of Wisconsin Extension, Madison, WI*.
14. Slater, J. G., H. A. Stone, B. T. Palermo and R. N. Duvall. 1979. *J. Pharm. Sci.*, 68:49.
15. Carstensen, J. T. 1981. In *Progress in Quality Control of Medicines*, P. B. Deasy and R. F. Timoney, eds., Amsterdam: Elsevier, pp. 97–112.
16. Ertel, K. and J. T. Carstensen. 1989. *Pharm. Res.*, 6, S.143.
17. Ertel, K. and J. T. Carstensen. 1990. *Int. J. Pharmaceutics*, p. 61.

7.8 PROBLEMS (CHAPTER 7)*

(1) A solid dosage form contains 100 mg of drug substance, and when formulated assays 1% moisture. It loses 1.5 mg of its strength in one year. Will it lose 3% in two years?

(2) If the product in Problem (1) contains 2% moisture, would it lose 3 mg in one year?

*Answers on pages 240, 241.

(3) If the product in Problem (1) contains 2% moisture and lost 4.5 mg in two years, what would be the bound moisture?

(4) If a 100 mg product like the one in Problem (1) lost 3 mg per year at 45°C and 6 mg per year at 55°C, what is the Arrhenius extrapolated stability (loss per year) at 30°C?

CHAPTER 8

Crystalline Solids

The morphology of a solid substance is of exceeding importance in its performance, both biologically and chemically, in a dosage form. Morphology simply implies "shape," and some discussion will be devoted to this concept.

8.1 MORPHOLOGICAL CONSIDERATIONS

Solids are either crystalline or amorphous [1]. A crystalline substance is characterized by having a crystal lattice, which is, in essence, a periodic array. If one were "positioned" on a molecule and progressed in a certain direction, one would encounter another molecule at a distance a, a second molecule at distance $2a$, etc. Likewise, in another principal direction, the distances would be b, $2b$, etc., and in a third direction they would be c, $2c$, $3c$, etc. a, b, and c are denoted the lattice constants. The angles between the directions can either be right angles or be oblique or sharp. The general classification of crystal systems [2] will be covered in this chapter.

An example of a crystal is shown in Figure 8.1. For the example to follow, it is assumed that $a = b = c$. If one wishes to have an idea of the order of magnitude of a of, for instance, aspirin, one may make the following calculation. Aspirin has a molecular weight of 180 and a solids density of 1.25 g/cm³, hence the molar volume is $180/1.25 = 144$ cm³/mole. There are $6 \cdot 10^{23}$ molecules in a mole, so that the volume of one molecule is $144/(6 \cdot 10^{23}) = 240 \cdot 10^{-24}$ cm³ $= 240$ Å³. If the molecule is a sphere contained in a cube (as shown in Figure 8.1), then the diameter of the cube is $(240)^{1/3} = 6.2$ Å, which would then be the molecular spacing. Distances between molecular layers can be found by X-ray diffraction (Figures 8.2 and 8.3). Two X-rays with a given wavelength, λ, are reflected from the

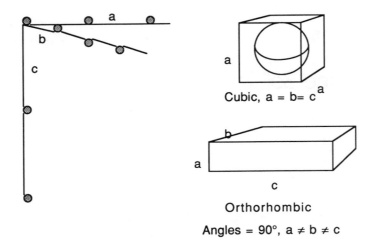

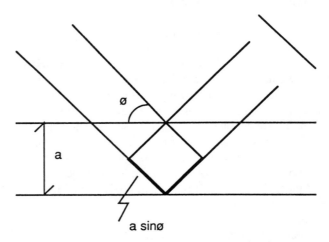

Cubic, a = b= c

Orthorhombic

Angles = 90°, a ≠ b ≠ c

FIGURE 8.1. *Example of crystal lattice.*

FIGURE 8.2. *X-ray hitting planes of molecules.*

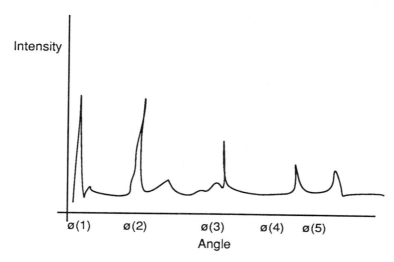

FIGURE 8.3. *X-ray diffraction pattern.*

crystal as shown, i.e., one is reflected from the surface and the other from the first molecular layer. The second wave traverses a distance that is $2 \cdot a \cdot \sin(\phi)$ longer than the first wave. If the two waves are in phase, they will reinforce each other and the signal will be amplified at the collimator (the collector, at the upper right in the figure). In the experiment, one changes the angle ϕ and the wavelength is fixed (and known). One notes the angles at which fortification occurs, and the extra distance in Figure 8.2 must therefore equal one wavelength, i.e.

$$2 \, [a \cdot \sin(\phi)] = \lambda \qquad (8.1)$$

so that all quantities except a are known. Reflection occurs from the second and subsequent layers as well, but their intensities are much lower. Actually the right-hand side of Equation (8.1) is (for general use) $n\lambda$. The X-ray pattern that emerges has the appearance shown in Figure 8.3.

The above refers to powder diffraction [3]. Single-crystal X-ray characterization will not only place the molecular positions in the lattice, but will also pinpoint the position of each atom [4,5].

Thermal methods (differential scanning calorimetry [6]) are also used as powerful tools in morphological investigations, and will be treated in the next chapter.

8.2 DRUG PURIFICATION

In the manufacture of solid dosage forms, the drug substance used must be as pure as possible. At the end point of the actual synthesis, it will contain impurities, and as many of these as possible must be removed. An *impurity* is distinguished from a *decomposition product*. The latter is a result of decomposition of the drug in the solid dosage form after manufacture. Impurities and decomposition products in certain cases can be the same substance, e.g., salicylic acid is an impurity in aspirin and is also the main decomposition product. Aspirin anhydride is, however, an impurity since it is not a decomposition product at room temperature.

It is worthwhile to review how a drug substance is purified. This occurs, on an industrial scale, primarily by two processes: recrystallization or precipitation. The principles are illustrated by example below.

Sulfanilamide [7] has the solubilities (Merck Index) shown in Table 8.1. If 40 g of sulfanilamide are allowed to dissolve in 1000 g of water at 60°C (and filtered if not all goes into solution) and the solution is allowed to cool to 25°C, then the amount of sulfanilamide that can be dissolved would be 7.5 g, so that approximately $40 - 7.5 = 32.5$ g of sulfanilamide would precipitate. The solubility of the impurities (present in small amounts) would most often not be superseded, so that the sulfanilamide crystals would be fairly pure. (Sometimes successive crystallizations are necessary.) If the cooling is slow, then the crystals are fairly large; if it is fast, then they are fairly small.

It might seem rather logical to make them small, since this would mean a large specific surface area, so that rapid dissolution would be favored, but there are adverse effects of small particles as well, such as poor flow and (in the case of tablets) capping tendencies. Hence a controlled particle size (giving the optimum of all properties) is usually what is required.

The purity of a drug substance can be determined by various means: (1) chemical assay (e.g., HPLC), (2) phase solubility, (3) differential scanning calorimetry, all giving quantitative results, and (4) by thin layer chromatography, giving qualitative results.

TABLE 8.1 Solubility of Sulfanilamide in Water [7].

Temp (°C)	Solubility g/1000 g Water
10	2.6
25	7.5
60	40

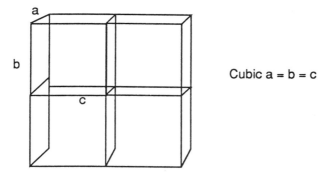

FIGURE 8.4. Cubic lattice. There is a molecule in each shown corner.

Precipitation is a purification mode [8] that is also best described by example. It is known that one gram of sulfanilamide dissolves in 5 cm³ of acetone at 10°C. If 95 cm³ of water are added, then the 100 cm³ are "almost" water, i.e., the solubility would be about 2.6 g/liter, i.e., 0.26 g in the ca 100 cm³ of solution. Hence $1 - 0.26 = 0.74$ gram of purer material would precipitate out. When a drug substance is purified in this fashion it is almost always very fine.

8.3 CRYSTAL SYSTEMS

There are seven different crystal systems [9,10]. For purposes here it is not necessary to know them, simply to be aware of their existence and in what respect they differ. In the cubic system (Figure 8.4), all sides in the lattice are equal and all angles are right. In referring to crystals in the following, the assumption will often be made (for simplicity) that the crystal in question is cubic. There is then the orthorhombic, where all the angles are 90° but the sides are unequal. In the monoclinic all sides are different, two angles are 90° but one is not. The remaining systems are combinations of non–right angles and sidelengths, and for completion are simply mentioned here: triclinic, tetragonal, trigonal, and hexagonal.

An inorganic compound will usually crystallize in a specific system. For instance, sodium and potassium chloride crystallize in the cubic system. There are exceptions (e.g., sulfur, which can be both rhombic and monoclinic). Organic compounds, however, invariably can crystallize in different crystal systems, depending on which solvent is used for recrystallization or which solvent pair is used for precipitation. This phenomenon is referred to as polymorphism [11,12]. This is very important pharmaceutically and will be the subject of discussion shortly.

8.4 CRYSTAL HABIT

Crystals from different crystal systems when viewed under the microscope will show different "faces." However, when viewed macroscopically, a different shape may not necessarily imply a different crystal system.

When a crystal precipitates from a supersaturated solution, the first event that occurs is the creation of a nucleus. This nucleus then grows (Figure 8.5). If growth is of equal rate in all directions, then a fairly cubical-looking shape will occur. If the growth is inhibited in one direction, then a plate will occur, and if it is inhibited in two directions, then a needle will be the result. Such shape differences do not imply different crystal systems, but are called crystal habits. They are important, since a cubic-like shape, for instance, will flow better in a powder hopper. This is important in tableting and encapsulation, as mentioned earlier. On the other hand, the less "cubic" a crystal becomes, the larger the specific surface area, so dissolution rates are favorably affected.

8.5 VAPOR PRESSURE OF SOLIDS

A solid is associated with a vapor pressure, which in most cases is small. Of pharmaceutical solids, two—nitroglycerin and ibuprofen—have measurable vapor pressures at room temperature.

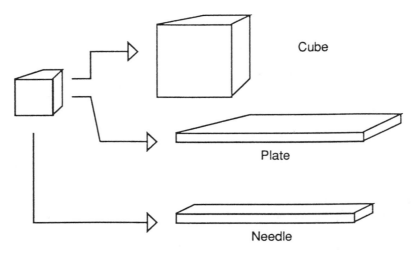

Cube

Plate

Needle

FIGURE 8.5. *Nucleus growth.*

TABLE 8.2 Vapor Pressure Data for Benzoic Acid.

Temp (°C)	1000/T (K⁻¹)	P (mm Hg)	ln P
25	3.354	0.0071	−4.948
45	3.14	0.0360	−3.324
65	2.96	0.150	−1.897
85	2.79	0.532	−0.631

Vapor pressures, P, will increase with absolute temperature, T, by the Clausius-Clapeyron equation:

$$\ln [P] = -\{\Delta H^*/R\}(1/T) + \beta \tag{8.2}$$

where H^* is the heat of sublimation, R is the gas constant, and β is a constant. Vapor pressure data for benzoic acid are listed in Table 8.2. These data are plotted in Figures 8.6 and 8.7.

Henry's law applies to a situation such as the one shown in Figure 8.8. A substance is present in the gas phase with a vapor pressure, P', and will partition between this and the liquid phase, where it will have a (molal) concentration C. Henry's law states that there is proportionality between these two quantities, with proportionality constant K:

$$C = KP' \tag{8.3}$$

This may be written:

$$\ln C = \ln [K] + \ln [P'] \tag{8.4}$$

If there is excess of solid present, the solution will be saturated. The vapor pressure of the compound will be its natural vapor pressure, P, so that we may write:

$$\ln [S] = \ln [K] + \ln [P] \tag{8.5}$$

All three quantities will change with temperature, K will change as

$$\ln [K] = -\{\Delta H^\P/R\}(1/T) + \beta'' \tag{8.6}$$

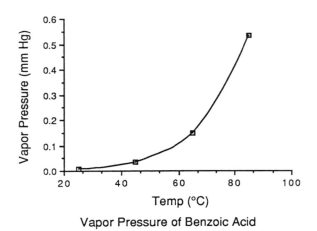

FIGURE 8.6. *The vapor pressure of benzoic acid as a function of temperature.*

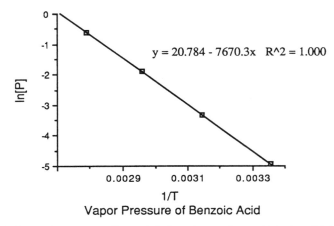

y = 20.784 - 7670.3x   R^2 = 1.000

FIGURE 8.7. *Data in Figure 8.6 plotted according to Equation (8.2).*

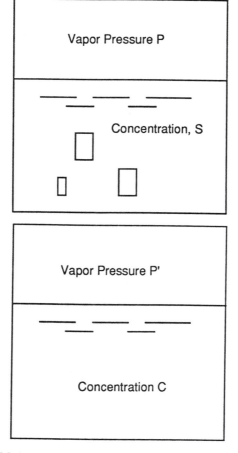

FIGURE 8.8. *Vapor pressures in saturated and over-saturated systems.*

and introducing this and Equation (8.3) into Equation (8.5) gives

$$\ln [S] = -\{\Delta H^*/R\}(1/T) + \beta - \{\Delta H^\P/R\}(1/T) + \beta''$$

$$= \ln [S] = -\Delta H/RT + q \qquad (8.7)$$

where ΔH is now the heat of solution.

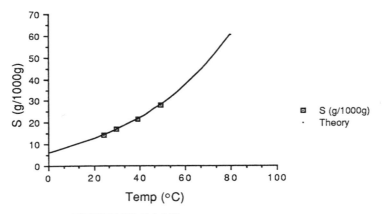

FIGURE 8.9. *Solubility versus temperature curve.*

8.6 SOLUBILITY MEASUREMENTS

Solubilities are determined by placing an excess of solid in contact with the liquid in question in a constant temperature bath and agitating the system for a sufficient period of time, so that the concentration of drug in solution is constant. Some problems, at times, exist because in some cases the drug may hydrolyze in solution, but we will assume at this point that this is not the case. The solubility will, of course, be a function of the temperature, and we will assume in the following that the solubility increases with increasing temperature. (This is most often the case. Notable exceptions: many calcium salts, and methyl cellulose, have decreasing solubility temperature curves.)

If solubility is measured versus temperature, then a curve such as the one shown in Figure 8.9 will result. An example of this (sulfanilamide in ethanol) is shown in the first two columns of Table 8.3.

The relation that exists between temperature and solubility is:

$$\ln [S] = Q - [\Delta H/(RT)] \tag{8.8}$$

where S is solubility and ΔH is the heat of solution of the compound in the liquid. R is the gas constant. Data presented in this form from Table 8.3 are shown in Figure 8.10.

The two last columns in Table 8.3 show the logarithms of S and the inverse absolute temperature values. The least squares fit values are correlation coefficient $= -0.992$, slope $= -2760$, and intercept $= 11.92$ so

$$\ln S = -2760/T + 11.92 \tag{8.9}$$

TABLE 8.3 Solubility of Orthorhombic Sulfanilamide in Ethanol [6].

Temp (°C)	S (g/1000g)	1/T	ln S
47.4	28.1	0.00312	3.34
40.3	21.4	0.00319	3.06
29.6	16.7	0.00330	2.82
24.1	14.2	0.00336	2.65

The heat of solution can be calculated from this:

$$\Delta H/R = 2760 \text{ K}, \quad \text{so } \Delta H_{\text{solution}} = 1.99 \cdot 2760 = 5500 \text{ cal/mole} \quad (8.10)$$

Example 8.1

If only the two first points in Table 8.3 are used, calculate the heat of solution.

Answer 8.1

The slope would be $(3.34 - 3.06)/(0.00312 - 0.00319) = -4000$, so that $\Delta H = 1.99 \cdot 4000 = 8$ kcal/mole.

8.7 POLYMORPHISM

If sulfanilamide is recrystallized from water it is orthorhombic (form II), whereas recrystallization from ethanol gives rise to a monoclinic form

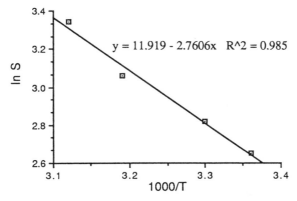

FIGURE 8.10. *Semilog-inverse treatment of data in Table 8.3 [Equation (8.8)].*

TABLE 8.4 Solubility of Monoclinic Sulfanilamide in Ethanol [6].

Temp (°C)	1/T	S (g/1000 g)	ln S
59.1	0.00300	31.5	3.45
58.8	0.00310	19.8	2.99
39.4	0.00319	14.0	2.64

Correlation coefficient −0.998, slope −4270, intercept −16.247.

(form I). The solubility of the orthorhombic sulfanilamide in ethanol is shown in Table 8.3; that of the monoclinic form is shown in Table 8.4, and the data will plot similar to Figure 8.10.

If the data from the two tables are plotted on a graph similar to the one in Figure 8.10, then *two* lines occur (Figure 8.13). The "highest" line implies that the substance has a "higher" solubility than the "lowest" line.

At, e.g., 50°C the monoclinic form is less soluble than the orthorhombic form. It should be noted that the dissolved molecules do not differ. They are sulfanilamide in both cases. In fact, if at 50°C the solution of orthorhombic sulfanilamide is allowed to stand for long times, then at one point monoclinic crystal will start precipitating out. In other words, the solution is supersaturated (i.e., actually unstable), and will tend to the stable system. Once monoclinic material starts precipitating, the entire system will eventually convert to this, the stable form (at 50°C). The important thing is that the supersaturated solution is stable for some time. Hence if

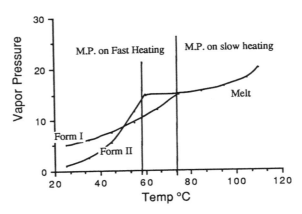

FIGURE 8.11. *Enantiotropic polymorphic pair.*

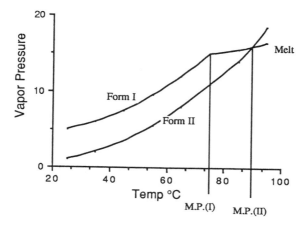

FIGURE 8.12. *Monotropic pair.*

a polymorph is more soluble than another, it will go into solution more quickly since

$$\text{Dissolution rate } = kA\,(S\,-\,C) \qquad (8.11)$$

and if S is higher in one case than in another, then the dissolution rate is higher too. The transition temperature in Figure 8.13 is 75°C.

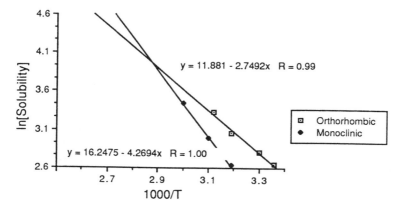

FIGURE 8.13. *Data from Example 8.2.*

8.8 METASTABLE SOLUTIONS

If water is cooled down very slowly and without agitation, it is possible to keep it liquid below 0°C for a while. Eventually ice will freeze out, but the metastable liquid state (the glass) can exist for varying lengths of time.

If an unsaturated solution of a substance is cooled to the point where it just becomes saturated, then precipitation will not occur. The temperature will have to be lowered further, and precipitation takes place from a super-saturated solution. The rate with which it takes place is a function of the substance, and of how undisturbed the system is kept.

In the previous example, if the "unstable" polymorph (in this case, at 50°C, the orthorhombic form) is kept dry, then it will not revert to the stable form, and it takes external influences such as pressure (e.g., in tableting) or moisture (as introduced in wet granulation) to effect a change of the crystal form.

If moisture is present then it will (in most cases) in time revert to the stable form. The reason for this is exemplified in Figure 8.14. If the metastable form is not stored at sufficiently dry conditions it will adsorb moisture. The moisture layer will saturate and the concentration will be S_2, the solubility of the metastable form. From the point of view of the stable polymorph, this, however, is a supersaturated solution, and eventually will start precipitating form I. Once some form I precipitates, the solution concentration will tend to decrease, but it then becomes unsaturated in form II, which will then dissolve in an attempt to keep the concentration at S_2. This

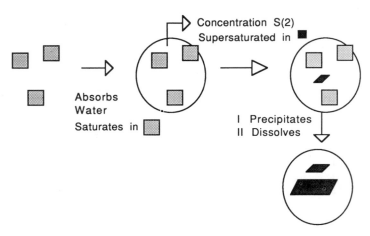

FIGURE 8.14. One mechanism whereby a metastable polymorph reverts to the stable species.

TABLE 8.5 Solubility of an Isoquinoline Derivative.

Temp (°C)	1/T	S (mg/mL)	ln S
60.3	0.00300	70	4.25
51.7	0.00308	50	3.91
31.9	0.00328	10	2.30
25	0.00336	2	0.69

will continue until all the II has been converted to I. But in the absence of moisture (or adsorbed moisture), form II is stable, and it is therefore not called unstable but rather it is referred to as a metastable polymorph. A polymorph can be metastable in the entire temperature region below the melting point, in which case the system is called monotropic (Figure 8.12). The situation can, however, occur where there is a transition point. Below a certain temperature, one form is metastable, above it is the stable form. In this case the system is called enantiotropic (Figure 8.11).

Equation (8.8) is of pharmaceutical advantage at 37°C, i.e., body temperature. The most soluble form at this temperature is the one that will give the highest *in vivo* dissolution, and it is therefore important to find out what the solubilities of various crystal forms are at different temperatures. This will be demonstrated by example.

Example 8.2

An isoquinoline exhibits the solubility behavior shown in Table 8.5. What conclusions can be drawn?

Answer 8.2

The data are plotted in Figure 8.15. It is seen that two lines occur, and that they intersect at $1/T = 0.003232$, i.e., $T = 1/0.03232 = 309.4$ K $= 36.24°C$. This is called the transition point. To the left of the transition point, form I will be more stable. The temperatures on the $1/T$ scale to the left of this point are temperatures higher than 36.24°C. Below this temperature the situation is reversed and form II is the more stable. Since 37°C is the temperature of interest—and since the most soluble is the advantageous form in a solid dosage form, from a biopharmaceutical point of view—the form that is metastable at 37°C is the form of preference in tablets and capsules, if the biopharmaceutical point of view is the determining one.

There have been cases in pharmaceutical history where this has been very important. For example, when the patent ran out on chloramphenicol,

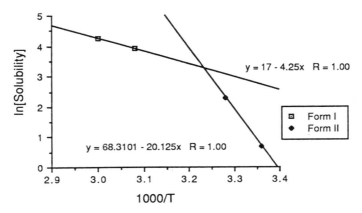

FIGURE 8.15. *Solubility plotting to determine a transition point.*

the innovators' products soon showed up to be more effective than the imitators' products. This was found to be due to the fact that the Parke Davis compound was a metastable polymorph with higher solubility, and therefore higher dissolution rates. The FDA, after this, instituted compulsory dissolution testing in ANDA's.

There are many cases where polymorphism is NOT important. If for instance the transition point is close to 37°C, as in Example 8.2, then the differences in solubility are only small. This for instance is the case with one of the polymorphic situations concerning ampicillin trihydrate. Hence, the

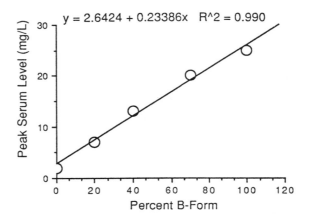

FIGURE 8.16. *Blood level peaks of chloromycetin palmitate. After Aguiar [13].*

mere existence of polymorphism is not sufficient to rule out sound use of generic equivalents.

It should be noted that the form that is metastable at 25°C (the usual storage temperature for pharmaceuticals in the U.S.) should NOT be used in ready-made suspension formulations since it will invariably convert on standing to the stable form, and this will give rise to crystal growth. It should also be mentioned that in nearly every case the amorphous form will be more soluble than the crystalline form (whether metastable or not).

8.9 EFFECT ON BIOPHARMACEUTICS

The interest in polymorphs in pharmaceutics historically has its origins in the fact that in the early 1960s, when chloramphenicol palmitate came off patent, several generic companies entered the market. It soon became evident that the generic preparations did not have the bioavailability of the innovator's (Parke Davis') product. Aguiar et al. [13] showed, as seen in Figure 8.16, that the peak blood level was a function of the amount of a metastable polymorph, i.e., in this case the product was more bioavailable because a metastable polymorph had been used. The product was a powder for reconstitution, and hence had had minimal physical impact in manufacturing before use, and is one of the few cases in pharmaceutics where a metastable compound is the one marketed. If possible, it would be desirable for this to be done in many other cases, since in general it implies increased bioavailability. However, the vicissitudes of manufacturing most often prohibit the use of any but the most stable polymorph known at the time.

This implies that the method is not foolproof. The most stable polymorph known at one point in time may not be the most stable polymorph. At a later point in time, accident may present the proper conditions for the formation of an even more stable polymorph. Roche, in the 1960s, was well into the clinical program with Valium™ when a more stable polymorph occurred by accident in the synthesis. In this case it was a monotrope, and it was never again possible to produce the less stable form used in the previous trials. Roche therefore had to repeat a large number of clinical studies.

8.10 REFERENCES

1. Carstensen, J. T. 1977. *Pharmaceutics of Solids and Solid Dosage Forms.* New York, NY: Wiley, pp. 1–3.

2. Kittel, C. 1956. *Introduction to Solid State Physics.* New York, NY: Wiley, pp. 9, 60, 478.

3. Suryanarayanan, R. 1989. *Pharm Res.*, 6:1017.
4. Pothisiri, P. and J. T. Carstensen. 1975. *J. Pharm. Sci.*, 64:1931.
5. Miyamae, A., S. Koda, S. Kitamoura, Y. Okamoto and Y. Morimoto. 1990. *J. Pharm. Sci.*, 79:189.
6. Guillory, J., S. Huang and J. Lach. 1969. *J. Pharm. Sci.*, 58:301.
7. Milosovich, G. 1964. *J. Pharm. Sci.*, 53:484.
8. Mullin, J. W. 1961. *Crystallization*. London: Butterworths, pp. 16–17.
9. Evans, R. C. 1966. *Introduction to Crystal Chemistry, Second Edition*. London: Cambridge U.P., pp. 32–35.
10. Martinez, H., S. F. Byrn and R. R. Pfeiffer. 1990. *Pharm. Res.*, 7:147.
11. Carstensen, J. T. 1980. *Solid Pharmaceutics, Mechanical Properties and Rate Phenomena*. New York, NY: Academic Press, pp. 14–19.
12. Haleblian, J. and W. McCrone. 1969. *J. Pharm. Sci.*, 58:911.
13. Aguiar, A. V., J. Krc, A. W. Kinkel and J. Samyn. 1967. *J. Pharm. Sci.*, 56:847.

8.11 PROBLEMS (CHAPTER 8)*

(1) A fairly water-soluble drug substance melts at 120°C. Aqueous solutions of it are stable. An excess of the drug is stirred in water for 96 hours at the temperatures shown below. Assume that in the event that a metastable polymorph had been used, it would all have been converted to the form that is stable at the temperature in question.

After 96 hours, samples are drawn from the supernatant and assayed, with the following results:

Temperature, °C	20	30	40	50	60	70
Solubility, g/100 g water	4	11	32	50	59.5	70

(a) Plot the solubility data in the proper fashion, and label the two polymorphs I and II, I being the form that is stable at 25°C.

(b) Which type of polymorphism is occurring (e.g., is it monotropism?)

(c) Determine the heat of solution for the two forms in cal/deg/mole (R = 1.99 cal/deg/mole).

(d) What is your estimation of the solubility of the compound at 80°C if determined in the manner shown above?

(e) If someone determined that their sample of the drug had a solubility, as determined above, of 75 g/100 g of water at 80°C what would your conclusion be?

*Answers on pages 241, 242.

(f) Which form would you utilize in a solid dosage form, if you desired a product stable to moisture, heat, and pressure during normal processing?

(g) Which form would be most bioavailable? (Assume that bioavailability is dissolution-dependent.) Explain why.

CHAPTER 9

DSC and Amorphates

In the previous chapter the crystalline state has been discussed. Measurement methods, which typically involve differential scanning calorimetry (DSC), will be discussed in this chapter. Aside from the crystalline state there is, as mentioned, also the amorphous state. This will be discussed below as well.

9.1 DIFFERENTIAL SCANNING CALORIMETRY (DSC)

The behavior upon heating of a solid is best studied by DSC. Hot stage microscopy is also useful. The use of thermal methods (DSC) in pharmaceutics is primarily due to the work of Guillory [1]. The principle of DSC is shown in schematic fashion in Figure 9.1.

Heat flows to a sample block of heat capacity $c(1)$ and to the sample $c(2)$, and the instrument splits the heat stream so that (in equilibrium) the amount of heat to the two entities is in the same ratio as the heat capacities, i.e., as the sample and control block heat up, they will have the same temperature. However, if a thermal event occurs in the sample (the block is inert, and is not subject to thermal events), e.g., melting, reaction, or dehydration, then extra heatflow or heat removal will be necessary, and this manifests itself in the form of a peak. In this text (as in many DSC instruments), a peak upwards is endothermic (such as melting or polymorphic transformation) and downwards is exothermic (i.e., the event is giving off heat, like crystallization).

The manner in which enantiotropes will behave is shown in Figure 9.2. It is noted that on slow heating, the transition has time to take place (the top DSC trace). After transformation, the crystal modification is form II, which then eventually melts [peak at $T(2)$].

151

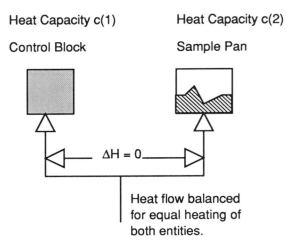

Heat Capacity c(1)   Heat Capacity c(2)

Control Block   Sample Pan

$\Delta H = 0$

Heat flow balanced
for equal heating of
both entities.

FIGURE 9.1. *Principle of differential scanning calorimetry.*

With fast heating, the transition can be bypassed, and the peak in the second DSC trace is the melting point of form I. However, above this temperature the melt is "supersaturated" in form II, and crystallization can occur (the exotherm in the last trace). After this, form II is present in solid form, and melts at $T(2)$ [peak at $T(2)$]. In the case of a monotropic pair (Figure 9.3) the top and the bottom are the straightforward melting point traces [peaks at $T(I)$ and $T(II)$]. However, the first trace leaves a melt at a tempera-

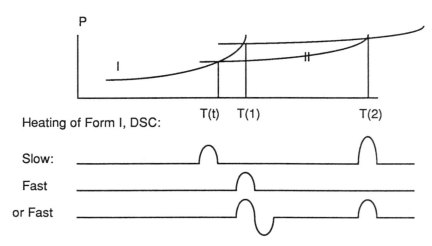

P

I

II

Heating of Form I, DSC: T(t)   T(1)   T(2)

Slow:

Fast

or Fast

FIGURE 9.2. *Behavior of an enantiotropic polymorph pair in a DSC.*

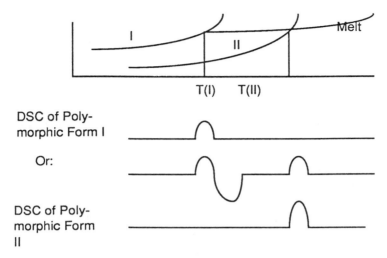

FIGURE 9.3. *Behavior of a monotropic pair in DSC.*

ture below $T(II)$. This is supercooled (with respect to form II) and this latter can crystallize out [the exothermic peak at $T(I)$ in the middle trace]. Above $T(II)$, in this case, form II is present, and melts at (the endotherm at) $T(II)$.

Heating rates in DSC are of importance. Figure 9.4 shows the melting point of extended-chain crystals of linear polyethylene as a function of heating rate [2].

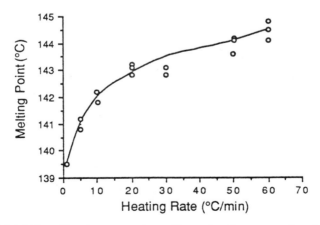

FIGURE 9.4. *Effect of heating rate on the melting point of a compound on the observed melting point.*

9.2 AMORPHATES

Materials that are not crystalline are amorphous. The best way of visualizing an amorphate is as shown in Figure 9.5.

If a molten substance is cooled slowly and without disturbing it, it is possible to supercool it (i.e., cool it below its melting point). If the liquid at this point is not very viscous, then it usually will not take much of a disturbance to make it precipitate out. An example of this is water. If cooled carefully, temperatures as low as $-20°C$ can be easily attained. However, the slightest stir will cause the ice to freeze out.

Crystallization rates are inversely proportional to viscosity, and if a substance is very viscous at its melting point, then supercooling becomes much easier. The "solid" thus formed is actually a liquid with very (infinitely) high viscosity. But even glass (which is mostly amorphous) is "liquid." Old church windows in Europe are thicker at the bottom than at the top, showing the flow with time.

If an appropriate property [e.g., heat capacity (Figure 9.5)] is plotted versus temperature, then there is a sharp break at the melting point for the crystalline compound. For the amorphate, however, there is no melting point, and there is a gradual transition at the so-called glass transition temperature (T^*). Above this temperature the amorphate retains the properties of a liquid (e.g. plastic deformation) and is denoted "rubbery." Below this temperature it has more of the properties of a crystalline solid [it can both deform plastically (like NaCl) or brittlely (like dicalcium phosphate) and is denoted glassy]. Chemical stability of rubbery amorphates is like the stability of the liquid (and is generally worse than that of the crystalline compounds [3]). Glass transition temperatures are often a function of moisture

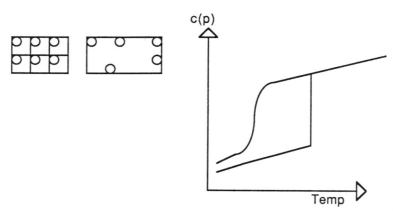

FIGURE 9.5. *Amorphate behavior as a function of temperature.*

content, e.g., PVP [4], which is of importance in granulations, since PVP is often used in wet granulation. If dried too far, the glass transition temperature may rise above room temperature, and the granule will be much more brittle, and often not compress.

9.3 SOLUBILITY AND AMORPHATES

In general, amorphates are less stable (more energetic) than crystalline substances (even the metastable polymorphs). The best way of visualizing their solubilities is by considering their moisture pickup at a given relative humidity. It can be shown [5] that these rubbery states are essentially supersaturated solutions. For instance, amorphous sucrose will pick up moisture at a given relative humidity to a point that is on the extension of the vapor pressure/concentration curve for sucrose solutions.

Example 9.1

At 32% RH amorphous sucrose will pick up 6 grams of water per 100 grams of amorphous solid. What is the solubility of a supersaturated sucrose solution representing the pseudo-equilibrium solubility of the amorphate in water at 25°C?

Answer 9.1

The "solution" contains 100 g of sucrose per 6 g of water, i.e., the "solubility" is $(100/6) \times 100 = 1666$ g of sucrose/100 g of water.

9.4 AMORPHOUS SUCROSE DOSAGE FORMS

There are dosage forms (pharyngets, candies) that are amorphous sucrose. At the onset they are "crystal clear," because they are not crystalline at all, but rather a glass. With time they will become turbid, because the glass is a supersaturated solution, and crystalline sucrose will precipitate out.

9.5 STABILITY OF AMORPHOUS SUBSTANCES

Amorphous solids usually decompose by first order kinetics [6,7]. It stands to reason that amorphous substances in general would be less stable than those in the crystalline state. This has been investigated by Morris [6] and Morris and Carstensen [3], who have shown that amorphous indomethacin exhibits stability that falls on the same line on an Arrhenius plot as that of the liquid melt. In the rubbery state, therefore, it is concluded that the amorphous state, in terms of stability, is simply an extension of the molten state. In the glassy state [7], however, the decomposition more resembles that of the crystalline solid.

9.6 POLYMERS

Polymers are an important group of solids, encompassing the natural polymers that have already been discussed (cornstarch for instance), and the synthetic ones (e.g., polyplasdone and polyethylene).

Mixtures of synthetic polymers are used at times, and polystyrene and poly(phenylene oxide) (denoted PPO) [8] is an example of such compatible blends—it forms clear films in binary mixtures and shows only one glass transition temperature [9], T^*. If the weight fractions of the two polymers are W_1 and W_2, then the so-called Fox equation [10] states that the glass transition temperature T^* of the blend will be given by:

$$1/T^* = (W_1/T_{g1}) + (W_2/T_{g2}) \tag{9.1}$$

where T_{g1} and T_{g2} are the individual glass transition temperatures. This has been shown to hold, e.g., for polyvinyl chloride and ethylene-vinyl acetate copolymers [11], and for polystyrene and PPO polymers as well [12–14].

Mixtures are, however, often not compatible. In such cases they will not form clear films, and the thermogram of the binary mixture will show two glass transition temperatures.

9.7 REFERENCES

1. Guillory, J. K., S. Huang and J. Lach. 1969. *J. Pharm. Sci.*, p. 58.
2. Wunderlich, B. 1973. *Macromolecular Physics: Crystal Structure, Morphology, Defects.* New York, NY: Academic Press.
3. Morris, T. 1990. Ph.D. thesis, U. Wisconsin, School of Pharmacy, Madison, WI 53706.
4. Oksanen, S. 1990. Master's thesis, U. Wisconsin, School of Pharmacy, Madison, WI 53706.
5. Carstensen, J. T. and K. VanScoik. 1990. *Pharm. Res.*, 25:1278.
6. Morris, T. 1990. Ph.D. thesis, U. Wisconsin, School of Pharmacy, Madison, WI 53706.
7. Pikal, M., A. L. Lukes and J. E. Jang. 1977. *J. Pharm. Sci.*, 66:1312.
8. MacKnight, W. J., F. E. Karasz and J. R. Fried. 1970. In *Polymer Blends, Vol. I*, D. R. Paul and S. Newman, eds., New York: Academic Press, p. 242.

9. Gedde, U. W. 1990. *Drug Dev. Ind. Pharm.*, 16:2465.

10. Fox, T. G. 1956. *Bull. Am. Phys. Soc.*, 1:123.

11. Hammer, C. F. 1971. *Macromolecules*, 4:69.

12. Blair, H. E. 1970. *Anal Calorim.*, 2:51.

13. Blair, H. E. 1970. *Polym. Eng. Sci.*, 10:247.

14. Prest, W. M. and R. S. Porter. 1972. *J. Polym. Sci., Polym. Phys. Ed.*, 10:1639.

9.8 PROBLEMS (CHAPTER 9)*

(1) In a drug substance that is monoclinic, if the wavelength of an X-ray is 1.5 Å, and peak angles of 4, 6, 8, and 9° are found, what are the corresponding spacings?

(2) A drug substance is amorphous, and exhibits a 1% loss after three years at 25°C (room temperature). The crystalline modification melts at 94.9°C and the melt, when tested for stability, exhibits first order decomposition with rate constants of 2.6% loss after one day at 95°C and 4% loss after one day at 99.85°C. Is the material in the rubbery state at room temperature?

*Answers on pages 242, 243.

CHAPTER 10

Hygroscopic Potential of Solids

There are two aspects to the concept of hygroscopicity [1–5]: (1) the potential for moisture uptake, and (2) the rate with which the moisture is taken up. This chapter deals with the former, i.e., the potential a solid substance has for water uptake.

10.1 WATER'S VAPOR PRESSURE

The vapor pressure of a pure compound is a function of temperature. Table 10.1 shows the vapor pressure, P', of water as a function of temperatures from $-40°C$ to the boiling point.

The Clausius-Clapeyron equation [1] states that the logarithm of the vapor pressure is linear in $(1/T)$, with a slope of $-\Delta H/R$, i.e.

$$\ln [P] = Q - \{\Delta H/R\}[1/T] \qquad (10.1)$$

If the data in Table 10.1 is plotted by the Clausius-Clapeyron equation (Figure 10.1), then two distinct lines result, one for the solid (ice) one for the liquid (water). In the latter case the slope of the line is

$$-5195.3 = -\Delta H/1.99$$

so

$$\Delta H = 10,338.6 \text{ cal/mole} = 10,338.6/18 = 574 \text{ cal/gram}$$

close to the 580 cal/gram usually reported as water's heat of vaporization.

TABLE 10.1 Water's Vapor Pressure at Different Temperatures.

Temp (°C)	Vapor Pressure (mm Hg)	1000/T	ln [P]
−40	0.10	4.92	−2.303
−30	0.29	4.12	−1.238
−25	0.48	4.03	−0.734
−20	0.78	3.95	−0.248
0	4.6	3.66	1.526
15	12.8	3.47	2.549
25	23.8	3.36	3.170
35	42.2	3.25	3.742
50	92.5	3.10	4.527
100	760	2.68	6.633

10.2 PHYSICALLY MOISTURE SENSITIVE DRUGS

Drugs are processed, packed, transported, and stored in a variety of environments. For instance the air may be more or less moist (humid), and the distinctions between a "humid" day and a "dry" day are well known.

Drugs may be (and often are) moisture sensitive. An example of where manufacturing of a dosage form is dependent on the humidity of the atmosphere is hard shell capsules. When the atmosphere is too moist (above 35% RH for even short exposures), the gelatin will pick up moisture, the shells will become sticky, and will not separate in the rings.

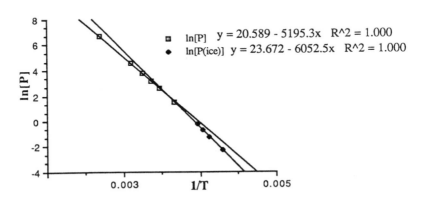

Water/Ice, plotted by Clausius-Clapeyron

FIGURE 10.1. Water/ice vapor pressures plotted by the Clausius-Clapeyron equation.

Another example is effervescent tablets. These are mixtures of sodium bicarbonate ($NaHCO_3$) and tartaric acid [$R(COOH)_2$]. When the tablet is added to water, the two will react:

$$2NaHCO_3 + R(COOH)_2 \rightarrow R(COONa)_2 + 2H_2O + 2CO_2 \quad (10.2)$$

This reaction must, however, not occur in the tablet, since if it does, then there will be no (or reduced) effervescence at the time the tablet is used. Since the reaction is catalyzed by moisture, and since it produces moisture, it will accelerate if it starts. Effervescent tablets are therefore produced in very low humidity areas, and packaged in aluminum foil (produced dry, and kept that way), or in tubes that will allow escape of water (allowing some reaction to take place, but allowing produced moisture to escape, so that the reaction will occur, but not accelerate).

10.3 RELATIVE HUMIDITY

It is apparent from the above that it is necessary to know, in a quantitative sense, how to describe humidity in the atmosphere (environment), and this is done through the well-known concept of relative humidity (RH).

If a room is 26°C and a sample of the air is taken in a closed container (Figure 10.2), and exposed to a strong desiccant (phosphorus pentachloride for instance), then the moisture in the air sample will be ad/absorbed and the pressure will drop because the moisture is now no longer in the gas phase. The pressure drop (say, e.g., 10 mm Hg) is the partial vapor pressure of the water (P) in the atmosphere from which the sample was taken.

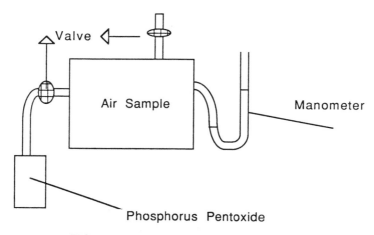

FIGURE 10.2. *Schematic for relative humidity.*

We express this quantitatively in this way. The vapor pressure could have been the saturation pressure, P (Table 10.1), i.e., 25 mm Hg, but it is only 10 mm Hg, so the pressure is $10/25 = 0.4 = 40\%$ of what it could be at most. So the relative humidity, RH, is 40%. In other words:

$$RH = 100 \, P/P' \qquad (10.3)$$

The relative humidity in a room can be measured by a sling psychrometer. This consists of two thermometers (Figure 10.3), one that is kept wet by means of a piece of wet gauze, one that is simply dry. When rotated rapidly, the water will start evaporating from the wet bulb. The drier the atmosphere is, the more rapidly the water in the gauze will dry, so that the "wet bulb temperature" will be low if the atmosphere is dry, and high if it is humid. Tables of conversion exist, so that the temperatures recorded can be converted into % RH (Table 10.2).

Example 10.1

If the dry bulb is 23.5°C and the wet bulb is 22°C, what is the RH?

Answer 10.1

In the middle of 92 and 84, i.e., at 88% RH.
RH is controlled on a large scale by air conditioning (or in slightly smaller rooms by dehumidifiers). The principle is illustrated by the following. If on

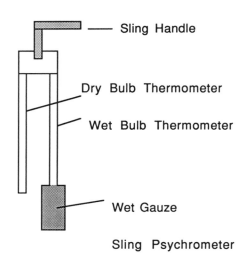

FIGURE 10.3. Principle of a sling psychrometer.

TABLE 10.2 Psychrometric Conversion Table.

Wet Bulb (°C)	Dry Bulb			
	21°C	22°C	23°C	24°C
20	91% RH	83% RH	76% RH	70% RH
21	100% RH	92% RH	84% RH	80% RH
22		100% RH	92% RH	84% RH
23			100% RH	92% RH

the hottest and most humid day of the summer it is 100% RH and 35°C, then (Table 10.1) the water vapor pressure is 42.2 mm Hg. Air is drawn into the air conditioner and cooled, e.g., to 15°C, where the vapor pressure is 12.8 mm Hg. This means that the air is supersaturated in water, and the excess water will condense. The condensed water is then removed physically. The air itself is then heated up to, e.g., 25°C (usual room temperature), in which case the RH now is

$$RH = 100 \, (12.8/23.8) = 54\% \text{ RH} \qquad (10.4)$$

since the saturation pressure at 25°C is 23.8. Sometimes, as in theaters and supermarkets, the air is not reheated, because the population in the rooms will heat up the air (and make it more humid by breathing). This is the reason why areas that are meant to hold crowds can be rather cold when no one is there.

Part of the storage life of pharmaceuticals is in well-controlled areas (manufacturing, and in the pharmacy itself), and there are usually 25°C and 40–60% RH. However, transportation of and warehousing can constitute environments much less favorable to the preservation of the dosage form.

10.4 VAPOR PRESSURES OVER IDEAL SOLUTIONS

Prior to discussing how to create rooms or spaces with controlled relative humidity, a short review will be given of vapor pressures over ideal solutions [2–5].

If two substances (e.g., water and acetone) form ideal solutions, and if V mL of water are added to $(100 - V)$ mL of acetone, then 100 mL of mixture of a volume % of $100 - V\%$ acetone is formed. Ethanol is a typical example of a substance that does not form an ideal solution with water, since when, e.g., 50 mL of water are added to 50 mL of ethanol, the resulting mixture will be less than 100 mL.

In an ideal mixture the vapor pressure of one component (e.g., water) will decrease from its pure vapor pressure (P_o) to P, given by

$$P = P_o[1 - x] \qquad (10.5)$$

where x is the mole fraction of the other component (e.g., acetone).

Example 10.2

What are the acetone and water pressures over a solution of 58% w/w of acetone in water? (Molecular weights are 58 and 18 respectively, and the vapor pressures of the pure substances are 300 and 25 mm Hg respectively.)

Answer 10.2

The number of moles of acetone in 100 g is $58/58 = 1$ mole. The number of moles of water is $42/18 = 2.33$ moles of water, i.e., 100 g of mixture is a total of 3.33 moles. Therefore the mole fraction of acetone is $X = 1/3.33 = 0.3$ so the mole fraction of water is 0.7. Hence,

- Water vapor pressure is $25 \times 0.7 = 17.5$ mm Hg.
- Acetone vapor pressure is $300 \times 0.3 = 90$ mm Hg.
- Total vapor pressure is 107.5 mm Hg.

If this is carried out under atmospheric conditions, the vapor pressure of air will be $760 - 107.5 = 652.5$ mm Hg.

The water, acetone, and total solvent vapor pressures over the entire concentration range are shown in Figure 10.4.

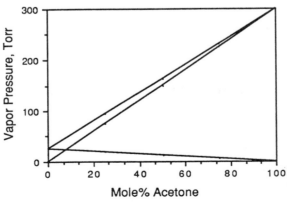

Vapor Pressure of Ideal Mixtures

FIGURE 10.4. *Vapor pressure mixtures of water and acetone, considering them (hypothetically) to be ideal mixtures.*

10.5 VAPOR PRESSURE OVER SALT SOLUTIONS AND SUSPENSIONS

The vapor pressure lowering alluded to previously is a so-called colligative property. It depends on the relative number of molecules in solution (hence the use of mole fraction). With an electrolyte, however, there will be ionization, e.g.

$$NaCl \text{ (solution)} \rightarrow Na^+ + Cl^- \tag{10.6}$$

Thus, for each mole of sodium chloride there will be not 6×10^{23} but 12×10^{23} molecular level "particles," i.e., to get Avogadro's number of molecules, not 58 but 29 g of sodium chloride are needed. One talks about this by stating that the equivalent weight of sodium chloride is 29.

If sodium chloride is dissolved in water, then the vapor pressure will decrease exactly in the same fashion as shown for, e.g., acetone. For instance, if 29 g of sodium chloride (one equivalent) are dissolved in 71 g of water $(71/18 = 3.94$ moles), then the equivalent fraction of sodium chloride will be:

$$X = 1/(1 + 3.94) = 0.2 \tag{10.7}$$

so

$$P/P_o = 1 - 0.2 = 0.8 \text{ or } 80\% \tag{10.8}$$

When solids are dissolved in liquids, however, there is one substantial difference: at a certain point, the solubility concentration is reached. If more solid is added, then it will simply stay there as a solid phase, and the vapor pressure will then be the same as that of a saturated solution. This is exemplified in Figure 10.5. Here it is shown that the solubility of sodium chloride in water at 25°C is 37 g/100 g solution. It is shown in the example below that the vapor pressure over this solution is 18.25 mm Hg, or 73% RH. If more sodium chloride is added it will not dissolve, and the water pressure will remain the same as for a saturated solution.

10.6 WATER VAPOR PRESSURE OVER AMORPHOUS SUBSTANCES

The aspects just mentioned apply to crystalline salt solutions. For non-ionizing crystalline materials, the same holds, and X is now simply the mole fraction of the solid. For amorphous materials the concepts are slightly different.

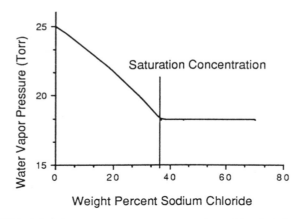

FIGURE 10.5. *Water vapor pressure over sodium chloride solutions.*

If a substance in the rubbery state is exposed to moisture, then it will take up moisture to a given level. This is shown in Figure 10.6. For instance, if the solid compound had a molecular weight of 360, and if it were exposed to a relative humidity of 60% ($P/P_o = 0.6$), then it might be determined (from weight increase) that 100 g of amorphate "adsorbed" 7 g of water. This corresponds to $100/360 = 0.278$ moles of amorphous drug and $7/18 = 0.39$ moles of water. If, instead of thinking of this as an adsorption, it is thought of as a supersaturated solution, then the concentration of drug

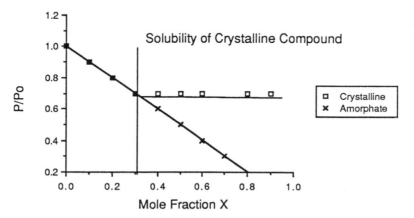

FIGURE 10.6. *Vapor pressure lowering of a crystalline versus an amorphous form of a compound.*

(in mole percent) would be $0.278/(0.278 + 0.39) = 0.42$. It is noted that this is consistent with the graph in Figure 10.6, where the vapor depression line is extended beyond the saturation point, and hence so-called "adsorbates" of amorphous materials are actually supersaturated solutions with sufficiently high viscosity to make them appear solid. VanScoik and Carstensen [6] have demonstrated this for sucrose.

10.7 CONTROLLED RELATIVE HUMIDITY

To test the behavior of drugs in various climatic conditions, it is necessary to be able to produce environments with known RH. This is done by means of saturated salt solutions, as shall be described below. It is recalled that in dilute (ideal) solutions, the vapor pressure of a solution, P, is related to the vapor pressure, P', of the pure solvent by the equation:

$$P/P' = 1 - X \qquad (10.9)$$

where X is mole fraction of solute. If the solution is saturated, the relation is only approximately true. In the case of aqueous solution, the term P/P', when multiplied by 100, is the RH [see Equation (10.3)].

Example 10.3

Sodium chloride has a molecular weight of 58, but dissociates into two ions when dissolved. It therefore has an equivalent weight of 29. It has a solubility of 37 g per 63 g of water (MW 18). What is the predicted relative humidity of a saturated solution?

Answer 10.3

37 g of NaCl $= 37/29 = 1.28$ equivalents, and 63 g of water is $63/18 = 3.5$ moles, so that $X = 1.28/(1.28 + 3.5) = 0.27$. Hence the RH over a saturated solution should be $100(1 - 0.27) = 73\%$, which is close to the actual figure (75%). The reason for the small deviation is that the solution is not ideal.

To create an atmosphere of 75% RH, one places a saturated solution of NaCl with an excess of NaCl (i.e., there are visible amounts of undissolved NaCl) in the bottom of a desiccator. When the desiccator is closed, the atmosphere will attain the vapor pressure of the saturated solution. Condensation or evaporation of water from the suspension on the bottom will not change the composition of the liquid (saturated) as long as there is solid present.

10.8 REFERENCES

1. Maron, S. H. and C. F. Prutton. 1965. *Principles of Physical Chemistry, Fourth Edition*. New York, NY: Macmillan, p. 78.

2. Carstensen J. T. 1977. *Pharmaceutics of Solids and Solid Dosage Forms*. New York, NY: Wiley, pp. 11–13.

3. Carstensen, J. T. 1980. *Solid Pharmaceutics: Mechanical Properties and Rate Phenomena*. New York, NY: Academic Press, pp. 131–133.

4. Carstensen, J. T. 1977. *Pharmaceutics of Solids and Solid Dosage Forms*. New York, NY: Wiley, pp. 8–11.

5. Carstensen, J. T. 1980. *Solid Pharmaceutics: Mechanical Properties and Rate Phenomena*. New York, NY: Academic Press, pp. 124–126.

6. VanScoik, K. and J. T. Carstensen 1990. *Pharm. Res.*, 7:1278.

10.9 PROBLEMS (CHAPTER 10)*

(1) Using a psychrometric table, determine the relative humidity in a room if the dry bulb temperature is 22.5°C and the wet bulb temperature is 20°C.

(2) Urethane has a molecular weight of 90 and a solubility at 25°C of 1 g per 0.5 g of water. What is the relative humidity over a suspension of urethane in water?

(3) Acetone (C_3H_6O) has a vapor pressure of 300 Torr and water a vapor pressure of 25 Torr. What is the water vapor pressure of a 58% by weight acetone solution?

*Answers on page 243.

CHAPTER 11

Pharmaceutical Packaging

Up until the mid-1950s, all pharmaceuticals were packaged in glass (except for cachets and products in tins). Glass is inconvenient because it is heavy (high transportation costs) and fragile. The advent of plastics, therefore, changed the profession and the industry.

One concern with plastics is the migration of substances from the plastic into the dosage form in the bottle. The nature and extent of such migrants (plastics additives) have been investigated by Kim et al. [1] and by Kim-Kang et al. [2]. The quantitative data of eight potential migrants in polyethylene terephthalate bottle walls [1] is listed in Table 11.1.

The authors point out [4–7] that the levels of phthalates are well below the levels of concern from a toxicological point of view [3]. In plastic bottles used for liquids, the migration of plasticizers and monomers into the solution is of primary concern. Although not to be disregarded, this is less prominent in solids because (1) the contact areas are much less, and (2) the fluidity of contact points are not nearly as amenable to permeation from one body to another. Migration might be expected where the vapor pressure of the plastics additive is significant. That this is not beyond the realm of possibility is evident in the daily observation of "plastic smells" (e.g., in new cars). These odors are usually not attributable to the polymer, but rather to some additive.

For the packaging of solids, the problem with plastics is that they allow permeation of moisture and oxygen, and for all practical purposes, this is not the case with glass. The discussion in the following will deal with this, and it will be assumed, in talking about bottles, that the seal is intact.

11.1 THE PHARMACEUTICAL CONTAINER-CLOSURE SYSTEM

The FDA guidelines refer to packages as container-closure systems. A typical bottle situation is shown in Figure 11.1. It should be noted that aside

169

TABLE 11.1 Potential Migrants in PET. Table Constructed from Data
Produced by Kim et al. [1].

Chemical Entity	Amount (mg/kg of PET)
Ethanediol 1,2	14
Terephthalic acid	20
bis-(2-ethylhexyl) phthalate	ca. 800
bis-(2-ethylhexyl) adipate	ca. 600
Dibutyl phthalate	ca. 200
Diethyl phthalate	ca. 100
Pyrogallol	ca. 1/2

from what is shown, the package as a whole also consists of a box and a
label insert, and each of these components contributes to the moisture protection of the product. Moisture permeation occurs (1) through the box, (2)
through the plastic itself, (3) through imperfections (cracks) in the plastic,
(4) through the seal, and (5) through imperfections in the seal.

11.2 MEASUREMENT OF MOISTURE PERMEATION

Moisture permeation through a bottle is determined by placing the bottle,
containing the dosage form, in an area with a defined relative humidity.
This could, for instance, be a desiccator with a salt suspension in the bottom well.

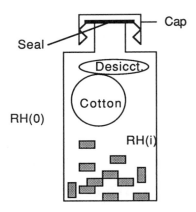

FIGURE 11.1. Schematic of bottle with components and dosage form.

TABLE 11.2 Moisture Pickup Rate.

Time (days)	Weight (g)	Moisture Pickup (mg/tablet)
0	150	0
1	150.05	0.5
2	150.1	1
4	150.2	2
8	150.4	4

The way in which the moisture permeation into a plastic bottle containing tablets is measured is exemplified below.

Example 11.1

A plastic bottle of thickness 1.0 mm contains 100 tablets each weighing 0.5 g. It is assumed that the air space over the tablets in the closed bottle has a zero RH. The bottle is now placed in a room that is 25°C and 75% RH. The bottle is weighed on an analytical balance daily. The results are shown in Table 11.2. The tare weight of the bottle and cap is 100 g. What is the amount of moisture penetrated per day per tablet?

Answer 11.1

The data are plotted in Figure 11.2. In general, such data give a slight lag time followed by a straight line. In the case presented here, the lag time is

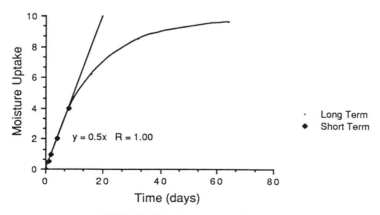

$y = 0.5x$ $R = 1.00$

· Long Term
● Short Term

FIGURE 11.2. *Data from Table 11.2.*

TABLE 11.3 Bottle from Table 11.1 Placed in Different RH-Environs.

Relative Humidity (percent)	Moisture Uptake Rate (mg/tablet/day)
50	0.33
75	0.5
100	0.67

not noticeable (i.e., the line goes through the point corresponding to the initial weight). The slope of the straight line is the moisture permeation rate. In this case it is seen from the data that this is 0.5 mg/tablet/day.

The moisture permeation rate is a function of (1) the plastic, (2) the thickness of the plastic, (3) the relative humidities inside and outside the package (and it is assumed here that it is zero inside), (4) the number of tablets within the bottle (i.e., how full it is), (5) the size (actually the surface area) of the bottle, and (6) how well it is sealed.

11.3 EFFECT OF RELATIVE HUMIDITY OF THE ENVIRONMENT

If a bottle of tablets or capsules is placed in a room, then the moisture exchange rate will be a function of the relative humidity of the room. The higher the relative humidity is, the higher the moisture uptake rate will be. This is exemplified in Table 11.3 and Figure 11.3. Figure 11.3 shows linearity

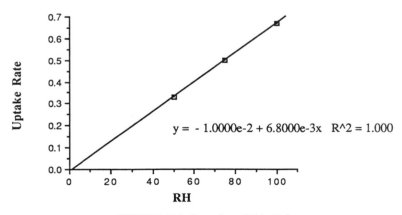

$y = -1.0000e-2 + 6.8000e-3x$ $R^2 = 1.000$

FIGURE 11.3. Data from Table 11.3.

with outside RH (RH_o). This is only true if the relative humidity inside the bottle (RH_i) is low, and can be assumed to be close to zero. It can be shown that the uptake rate is proportional to

$$Rate \approx RH_o - RH_i \tag{11.1}$$

Example 11.2

If, in Example 11.1, the external atmosphere had had a moisture of 50%, what would the moisture permeation rate have been?

Answer 11.2

The rate would have been $(50/75) \times 0.5 = 0.33$ mg/tablet/day.

11.4 EFFECT OF THICKNESS OF THE BOTTLE

It stands to reason that if a bottle is made thicker, then it will protect better against moisture, i.e., the moisture permeation rates will decrease with thickness. Figure 11.4 shows the bottle in Example 11.1, at the same conditions (25°C/75% RH) but with varying thicknesses of bottle. It is noted that the moisture permeation rate decreases, but not linearly. In fact, the moisture permeation rates are inversely proportional to the thickness of the bottle (Figure 11.5).

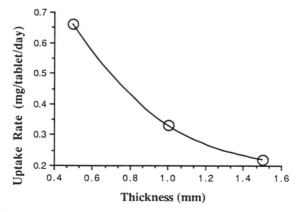

FIGURE 11.4. *Moisture uptake rate as a function of bottle thickness.*

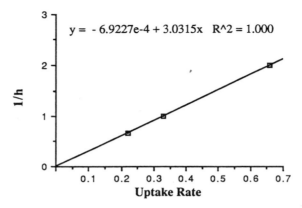

FIGURE 11.5. *Graph showing inverse proportionality between moisture uptake rate and bottle thickness.*

Example 11.3

What would the rate have been if the thickness of the plastic was 1.5 mm and the outside humidity 50% RH?

Answer 11.3

The rate would have been $(1/1.5) \times 0.33 = 0.22$ mg/tablet/day.
It was mentioned in Chapter 6 that drugs may be moisture sensitive.

Example 11.4

A tablet weighs 1.0 g and has a critical moisture content of 3 mg water per gram of tablet. It is produced at a level of 1 mg water per gram of tablet and packaged into a bottle containing 100 tablets. The bottles are 0.8 mm thick, which allows a permeation of 0.5 mg of water per day. How long will the product be satisfactory?

Answer 11.4

The largest amount the 100 tablets may absorb is $(3 - 1) \times 100 = 200$ mg of water. The bottle will allow permeation of this amount in

$$200/0.5 = 400 \text{ days}$$

11.5 THE GENERAL DIFFUSION EQUATION

It is seen from the previous examples that the moisture permeation rate can be obtained by plotting weight as a function of time. The rate with which moisture permeates a plastic bottle (excluding seal considerations) is given by:

$$\text{Overall rate} = D \times \text{Bottle surface area} \times (RH_{outside} - RH_{inside}) \quad (11.2)$$

$$\text{Rate per tablet} = \text{Overall rate/Number of tablets} \quad (11.3)$$

D is a permeation constant. These equations are useful because they make it possible to calculate the correct dimensions (thickness) of a bottle for use in a pharmaceutical product.

D is small for high-density plastics. It gets larger if there are "holes" in the plastic (e.g., created by large percentages and poorly dispersed pigments such as titanium dioxide). So if two bottles are made of the same plastic and general composition, and have the same dimensions, but one is opaque (contains opacifier such as titanium dioxide), then the opaque bottle is more permeable. D gets smaller the thicker the bottle is. In fact D is inversely proportional to the bottle thickness, h (mm):

$$D = Q/h \quad (11.4)$$

where Q is a constant.

The means of testing a tablet product in a bottle regarding its potential for moisture pickup is to place it in several atmospheres of different humidity (desiccators, for instance), with different RH values, and to monitor the weight gain as a function of time. From this it is possible to determine the rate with which the tablets in the bottle pick up moisture. If a particular rate is desired, then it is possible to calculate, e.g., how thick the bottle must be, since D is inversely proportional to the thickness.

Example 11.5

It is desired that the package shelf life be three years for the product in Example 11.4. How much thicker would the package have to be made to allow for this? (The term shelf life is used here in the approximate, non-statistical sense.)

Answer 11.5

Three years is 1100 days, so that the thickness would have to be increased by a factor of 1100/400 = 2.7. Since the thickness of the bottle in Example 11.4 was 0.8 mm, a thickness of 2.2 mm would be needed to accomplish a three-year package dating.

The diffusion equation, as mentioned, can be written [from Equations (11.2) and (11.3)]:

$$dm/dt = (D/h)\{P_o - P_i\} \qquad (11.5)$$

where m is the amount of moisture transferred. Both P_o and D are functions of absolute temperature, T, by an Arrhenius-type equation, i.e.

$$\ln [D] = A - (\Delta H_D/RT) \qquad (11.6)$$

and

$$\ln [P_o] = B - (\Delta H_p/RT) \qquad (11.7)$$

where A and B are constants, and where (ΔH_D) and (ΔH_p) are enthalpies of activation for the two parameters. Hence, the initial, linear portion of the diffusion process will give $(dm/dt)_{initial}$ which will be proportional to D and P_o, and hence:

$$\ln [(dm/dt)_{initial}] = (A + B) - \{(\Delta H_D + \Delta H_p)/RT\} \qquad (11.8)$$

The initial moisture uptake rates can therefore be assessed by such experimentation, but in general too many variables are at play, and the approach of one accelerated test (the Joel Davis test), viz. 40°C and 75% RH for 3 months, is the practice followed by industrial investigators. It is noted that for a product to stand up well under such conditions, a lot of factors have to be satisfactory (e.g., adhesion in film-seal).

11.6 EFFECT OF BOTTLE SIZE

The effect of bottle size is actually complicated, but the exact treatment does not give results greatly different from the following treatment. If the bottle size in Example 11.1 originally had been 100 mL, and was then changed in one experiment to 200 mL and in a third experiment to 300 mL, then the results might be as shown in Table 11.4 and Figure 11.6.

TABLE 11.4 Tablets from Example 11.1 in Different Bottle Sizes.

N = 100, W = 0.5 g/tablet, 25°C/75% RH, h = 1.0 mm		
Bottle Size (cm³)	Moisture Uptake Rate (mg/tablet/day)	6 × [Bottle Size]²ᐟ³ (area, cm²)
100	0.5	129
200	0.79	205
300	1.04	269

If it is assumed that the surface area is a shape factor (e.g., 6, as for the case of a cube) times $[Volume]^{2/3}$, then the results in the third column of Table 11.4 and in Figure 11.7 are produced.

Example 11.6

It is desired to change the bottle (but not the number of tablets), in the bottle in Example 11.1. The volume is increased by 50%, i.e., it is 1.4 times what it was originally. It is assumed that the surface area of the plastic is increased by the 2/3 powder of this amount. What would be the predicted moisture uptake rate?

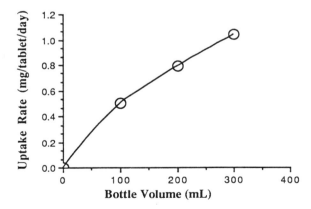

FIGURE 11.6. *Effect of bottle volume on uptake rate per tablet in a bottle with constant quantity of tablets.*

Answer 11.6 (See Figure 11.7)

The new volume, V', is 1.4 times the old volume, V. The new area, A', is $(1.4)^{2/3} = 1.25$ times the old area, A. 1.25 of 0.5 mg/day/tablet $= 0.63$ mg/day/tablet.

This is an interesting observation, because, e.g., if tablets are dispensed from a large bottle in a pharmacy, as it gets emptier, the uptake rate per tablet increases. However, relative humidities in pharmacies are well controlled and there is usually no problem in this sense.

It also has some bearing on the use of prescription bottles, but here the storage period is usually short (e.g., two weeks). The storage conditions in the average home are adverse to stability, since medication is usually stored in the medicine cabinet, which most often is right next to the shower. This is one of the reasons that patients should only take the medication during the prescribed period of time (and, e.g., not reuse a partly used prescription one year after it was issued).

It has been assumed above that when the tablets are in the bottle and when it is closed, an equilibrium sets up immediately with moisture in the tablet. This is obviously not true, and there is not always an equilibrium where there is a given moisture content in the atmosphere above the solid at a given content of moisture in the solid or the dosage form. This is a highly complicated situation and will not be treated here.

11.7 USP CONTAINER PERMEATION TEST

The considerations above only account for the problem of moisture permeation of the plastic. The seal, of course, may be defective as well. If

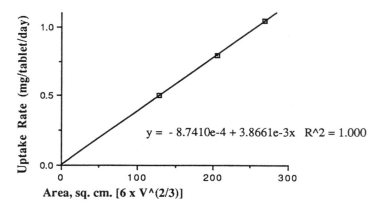

FIGURE 11.7. Uptake rate as a function of surface area of bottle.

one had an excellent bottle with a poor seal, nothing would be gained, so the USP method tests for both at the same time. The method is to be found in USP 20, p. 954, and in essence is as follows:

(1) Four mesh (i.e., rather coarse) calcium chloride is dried at 110°C, and is the desiccant to be used in the bottle.

(2) Twelve containers are selected, and they are opened and closed ten times.

(3) Ten of the containers are filled to 13 mm below the cap with desiccant and closed with a controlled torque. The two controls are filled with glass beads and similarly closed.

(4) The bottles are weighed to the nearest mg for a bottle smaller than 200 mL and to the nearest 10 mg for a larger bottle.

(5) The bottles are stored at 20°C for fourteen days at 75% RH and the weight determined. The volume of the bottle is determined at this point.

(6) The uptake rate (in mg/day/liter) is calculated from the difference in weight gain of the bottle from that of the control.

(7) The bottle is tight if no more than one bottle has picked up more than 100 mg/day/liter and none more than 200 mg/day/liter.

Example 11.7

A type USP tightness test is performed on a 50 mL package. The worst moisture pickup rate at 75% RH and 20°C for ten bottles in five days was 22 mg. Can the container be classified as being tight?

Answer 11.7

The moisture pickup rate was 22 mg/5 days/50 cc bottle = 4.4 mg/day/50 cc bottle = (1000/50) × 4.4 = 88 mg/day/liter which is less than 100 so that the bottles pass the test.

Example 11.8

Suppose that nine bottles had had less of a pickup than 22 mg, but that the tenth had picked up 55 mg. Would the container still be classified as tight?

Answer 11.8

Nine of the bottles pass, but the tenth must have a rate of less than 200 mg/day/liter. $(55/5) \times (1000/50) = 220$ mg/day/liter which is too high, so that the batch of containers cannot be classified as tight.

It is noted that the USP test is a classification test, and in case of particular products, a container that is classified as tight may not be adequate. See, for instance, Example 11.5.

11.8 STABILITY AND PACKAGING

A glass bottle with an adequate seal will protect the drug product inside from oxygen and moisture. Glass, however, is expensive and fragile. It also makes for a heavy product, so that transportation costs are high. It is for this reason a less optimal package, and the plastic package is opted for. In this, the product must be sufficiently stable so that expiration periods will be adequate.

It should be pointed out that none of the plastics on the market are complete barriers for oxygen, and that, therefore, if a product *is* packaged in glass, then the drug substance is probably somewhat oxygen-sensitive.

From the point of view of moisture, it has been shown earlier [Chapter 7, Equation (7.9)] that a product usually has a critical moisture content, a^*. Beyond this, the product will be much less stable, and as an approximation one may assume that the product is satisfactory if the moisture content is below a^*, and unsatisfactory if the moisture content is above.

Example 11.9

100 tablets are packaged in a bottle and the assembly allows a moisture permeation of 0.5 mg/day. The tablets weigh 0.7 grams apiece, and the initial moisture content is 0.5%. The critical moisture content is 0.8%. How long will the product be satisfactory?

Answer 11.9

There are 70 grams of tablets in the bottle. The allowable moisture uptake is $0.8 - 0.5 = 0.3\%$, i.e., 0.21 g or 210 mg. Since 0.5 mg of moisture penetrates per day, this corresponds to 420 days. Kim et al. [1] give the following

approximate moisture permeabilities of three different batches and manufacturers of PET containers: 23 ± 2, 30 ± 1, and 34 ± 2 mg/liter/day,
and correctly note that they all pass the USP test for tightness.

If the critical moisture content is arrived at after $t*$ days, then beyond this
point in time, the rate constant $k*$, will be a function of moisture content by:

$$k* = k' + qV \tag{11.9}$$

where q is a constant (solution rate constant times solubility), and V is the
amount of moisture present at time t. This, to an approximation is linear in
time, i.e.

$$V = Qt' \tag{11.10}$$

where t' is the time elapsed after the critical moisture content has been
reached, i.e.

$$t' = t - t* \tag{11.11}$$

Combining Equations (11.9) and (11.10) gives:

$$k* = k' + (qQ)\, t' = k' + At' \tag{11.12}$$

where

$$A = Qq \tag{11.13}$$

It is recalled from Chapter 7 that the decomposition is zero order and is
given by:

$$dM/dt' = -(k' + At') \tag{11.14}$$

which integrates to:

$$M = M_o - k't - (A/2)t'^2 = M_o - k'(t - t*) - (A/2)(t - t*)^2$$

$$= M_o - at - bt^2 \tag{11.15}$$

where a and b are constants. This situation, hence, leads to a decomposition
profile that is a parabola with downwards curvature. An example of this is
shown in Figure 11.8.

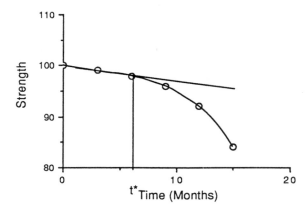

FIGURE 11.8. *Decomposition profile of drug product where the critical moisture content has been reached after six months.*

11.9 REFERENCES

1. Kim, H., S. G. Gilbert and J. B. Johnson. 1990. *Pharm. Res.*, 7:176.
2. Kim-Kang, H., S. G. Gilbert, A. W. Malick and J. B. Johnson. 1990. *J. Pharm. Sci.*, 79:120.
3. Thomas, J. A., T. D. Darby, R. F. Wallin, P. J. Garvin and I. Martis. 1978. *Toxicol. Appl. Pharmacol.*, 45:1.
4. Gilbert, S. G. 1975. *Env. Health Perspec.*, 11:47.
5. Gilbert, S. G. 1979. *J. Food Sci.*, 33:63.
6. Gilbert, S. G. 1979. *J. Food Qual.*, 2:251.
7. Koros, W. J. and Hopfenberg, H. G. 1979. *Food Technol.*, 33:56.

11.10 PROBLEMS (CHAPTER 11)*

(1) The moisture permeation of different bottles of the same plastic is considered. Consider the bottles simply to be cylinders. One bottle, A, has a diameter of 5 cm and a height of 10 cm. Another bottle, B, has a diameter, d, of 4 cm and a height, h, of 8 cm. The moisture permeation of bottle A is, initially, 0.5 mg/day. How much would it be for bottle B?

(2) In the USP tightness test, the moisture uptake is calculated as mg/day/liter. What does this presume as an assumption, and how would this calculate out for the figures in Problem (1)?

*Answers on pages 243, 244.

CHAPTER 12

Equilibrium Moisture Content of Solids

The problem of hygroscopicity is of importance in pharmaceutics. If a drug product is to be made, and if it is known that it is moisture-sensitive, then obviously it cannot be allowed to pick up large amounts of water during processing. The use of air conditioners is widespread, but capacities of such systems vary. The important aspect is to know how much moisture a solid substance will pick up at given conditions and to then assess how to change the surroundings so as to keep the quality of the drug product intact or optimum.

12.1 HYGROSCOPICITY

Hygroscopicity is the potential for moisture uptake that a solid will exert in combination with the rate at which this will happen. The condition of the atmosphere is an important factor as well, so a short, concise definition of hygroscopicity is not possible.

If a solid is placed in a room, then moisture will condense onto it. If this moisture occurs simply as a limited amount of adsorbed moisture, then the substance is not hygroscopic under those conditions. These conditions exist if the water vapor pressure in the surrounding atmosphere is lower than the water vapor pressure over a saturated solution of the solid in question.

Often, however, the water vapor pressure in the atmosphere, P_a, is higher than that of the saturated solution, P_s. If this is so, there will be a thermodynamic tendency for water to condense upon the solid. This is depicted in Figure 12.1.

It can be shown that the amount of moisture, W, which adsorbs is a function of time, t, of the vapor pressures in the atmosphere, P_a and P_s, and of

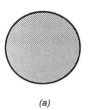   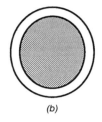   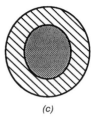

(a)   (b)   (c)

FIGURE 12.1. *Mechanism of moisture condensation. (a) Solid, (b) water condenses if*
$P_s < P_a$, *and (c) water layer saturates in drug substance.*

a mass transfer coefficient, k, by the following equation:

$$[W + B]^{1/3} = [k(P_a - P_s)E]t + [B]^{1/3} \qquad (12.1)$$

where

$$B = M_o \cdot C \qquad (12.2)$$

$$C = d*/d \qquad (12.3)$$

$$E = N^{1/3}\pi^{1/3}(6/S*)^{2/3} \qquad (12.4)$$

Here, N is the number of particles in the sample, d, is the density of the
solid and $d*$ is the density of a saturated solution of the solid in water. The
solubility is S g of solid/g of water. The integrating factor is predicated on
the assumption that there is no liquid layer ($W = 0$) at the onset ($t = 0$) of
the experiment. M_o is the initial amount of solid.

It is noted that from a thermodynamic point of view, the situation shown
dictates that moisture keeps on adsorbing until all solid has dissolved, and
then continues until the solution is sufficiently dilute to have a vapor
pressure of P_a. In this respect, the moisture uptake curve differs from that
of surface adsorption (polymers, and situations at atmospheric pressures
below P_s) because these asymptote at much lower levels.

Suppose a solid is placed in a room of a given RH, as shown in Figure
12.2. If the RH were 30%, then it might pick up moisture at a given rate, at
50% RH at a higher rate, and at 80% RH at an even higher rate.

The rate at which it picks up moisture is determined by weighing the sample at given intervals, as demonstrated in Table 12.1. It is noted that there is
a linear section of the curve (up to six days), as shown in Figure 12.3. The
slope of this linear segment is the MUR. The actual uptake rates (deter-

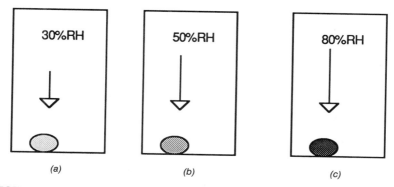

FIGURE 12.2. *Data from Table 12.2: (a) 0.083 mg/g/day; (b) 0.125 mg/g/day; and (c) 0.5 mg/g/day.*

mined from the linear portions) for 10 g samples of a solid are shown in Table 12.2.

The uptake rates can simply be obtained by weighing the sample after a given time (six days) but in such a case it is assumed that the moisture uptake is still in the linear phase. If for instance, the weight gain is 5 mg per 10 g sample in six days, then the MUR is $5/(10 \times 6) = 0.083$ mg/g/day.

If the MUR values are plotted versus RH, then a straight line results (Figure 12.4). It is noted that the curve intercepts the x-axis at 20% RH. This means that the compound can be stored without moisture pickup in atmospheres of less than 20% RH. In some cases the compound will dry out under such conditions (e.g., a hydrate), but in general the useful informa-

TABLE 12.1 Moisture Uptake of
Choline Bitartrate [1] at 50% RH.

Days Stored at 50% RH	Moisture Pickup mg/10 g
1	2.5
2	5
4	10
6	15
18	22.5
36	34
72	39.5
144	42
288	43

TABLE 12.2 Moisture Uptake Rate
of Choline Bitartrate [1].

% RH	mg/10 g/6 days	mg/g/day
30	5	0.083
50	15	0.25
80	30	0.50

tion gained from such a graph is the maximum RH that is satisfactory for storage of the product. Twenty percent RH happens to be the relative humidity over a saturated solution of the compound (or over a salt pair, as shall be discussed presently).

12.2 EQUILIBRIUM MOISTURE CURVES FOR SALT-HYDRATES

The previous section dealt with the *rate* with which moisture is taken up. As shown in Figure 12.3, at longer time periods, the moisture level (the weight of the sample) will taper off and plateau at an equilibrium value. This equilibrium value is also a function of RH, and there are two types of curves that occur when equilibrium values are plotted against RH — salt-pairs and continuous adsorption. The former will be discussed first.

For inorganic compounds and hydrates, the curves are stepwise curves. For instance, for disodium hydrogen phosphate, the following situation exists. The compound can form three hydrates (2, 7, and 12) aside from being

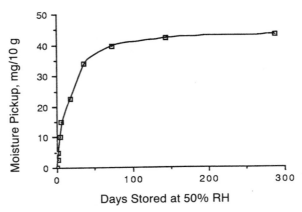

FIGURE 12.3. Moisture uptake of choline bitartrate at 50% RH.

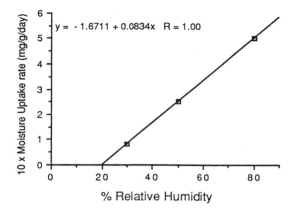

FIGURE 12.4. *Moisture uptake rate as a function of RH.*

anhydrous. The percent of moisture in, e.g., the dihydrate, is calculated as follows: disodium hydrogen phosphate has a molecular weight of 142. The dihydrate hence has a molecular weight of $142 + 36 = 178$. Hence, the moisture percentage is $100 \times (36/178) = 20\%$. The moisture contents for the remaining hydrates are shown in Table 12.3.

It is seen in the table that the relative humidity of the atmosphere above a mixture of anhydrous disodium hydrogen phosphate and the dihydrate is 9 mm Hg or $100 \times (9/24) = 38\%$ RH. It is noted that any mixture of the anhydrous salt and the dihydrate will give this relative humidity. Hence, disodium hydrogen phosphate containing between 0 and 20% moisture will have above it an atmosphere of 38% RH. Similarly, as shown in the table, the heptahydrate contains 47% moisture and mixtures of di- and heptahydrate give rise to water vapor pressures of 14 mm Hg (58% RH). Proceeding in this fashion, a graph as shown in Figure 12.5 results [1].

Two further points need to be mentioned. (1) If disodium hydrogen phosphate dihydrate is stored at a RH between 38 and 58%, it will not pick up

TABLE 12.3 Characteristics of Disodium Hydrogen Phosphate.

Type	% Moisture	P (Water)		RH
Anhydrous	0	Pair	9	38
Dihydrate	20	Pair	14	58
Heptahydrate	47	Pair	18	75
Dodecahydrate	60	Pair	22	92
Satd. solution				
(100 g water/4.5 g salt)				

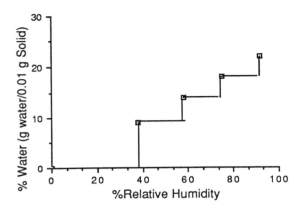

FIGURE 12.5. *Vapor pressure diagram of sodium phosphate.*

moisture. Once the relative humidity is raised to (slightly above) 58%, then it will start picking up moisture until it has completely converted into the heptahydrate. (2) If the relative humidity is raised to (slightly above) 92% RH, then the dodecahydrate is converted to saturated solution. At higher RH values, the equilibrium will be dictated by the water vapor pressure over the now unsaturated solution [see Equation (10.5) where X is mole fraction of solute].

At 100% RH the system in equilibrium is infinite dilution (pure water), and if a diagram such as this is carried out to 100% RH, then a sharply increasing curve should result at very high RH.

The diagram in Figure 12.5 involves a given temperature. Figure 12.6 shows a diagram of a dihydrate at different temperatures. At the temperature T_3 the line for the salt-pair has "caught up" with that of the saturated solution. Essentially this means that the enthalpy of hydration for the solid is higher than the heat of vaporization of water from the saturated solution, since both have Clausius-Clapeyron type vapor pressures. Above T_3, therefore, the salt would have a higher vapor pressure than the saturated solution, but this is thermodynamically untenable, and T_3 is simply the highest temperature (and a triple point) where the dihydrate exists.

TGA (thermal gravimetric analysis) or DSC are frequently used in the investigation of salt hydrates, e.g., cefaclor dihydrate [2]. In DSC it is shown that smooth desolvation begins at 64°C and that half of the water was lost at 74°C. The total water was lost at 110°C. In DSC there will be a varying relative humidity in the pan (which is usually punctured) and the only definitive statement that can be made in such a case is that 110°C is the critical temperature, above which the dihydrate does not exist.

12.3 EQUILIBRIUM MOISTURE CONTENTS FOR MACROMOLECULES

For an organic compound such as starch, a smooth equilibrium moisture curve will result. Here again there is the sharp upswing at very high relative humidities.

If experiments such as those exemplified in Table 12.1 and Figure 12.3 are carried out on, e.g., cornstarch, then curves of the *type* shown in Figure 12.7 result. The figure shows moisture uptake rate curves at four different relative humidities: 20%, 40%, 60%, and 80%. When the moisture contents (X mg water/mg solid) of these levels are plotted as a function of relative vapor pressure, P/P^* (the relative humidity, divided by 100, the so-called water activity) then an isotherm results. This moisture isotherm has the shape shown in Figure 12.8.

When $P/[X\{1 - P\}]$ is plotted versus P, then a straight line results (Figure 12.9).

12.4 ADSORPTION ISOTHERMS OF SILICA

It is noted that Figure 12.3 demonstrates that the equilibrium level is a function of the relative humidity at which the experiment is carried out. Figure 12.7 shows an example of moisture uptake curves of a 100 mg sample of silica, at various relative humidities. These levels are tabulated in the

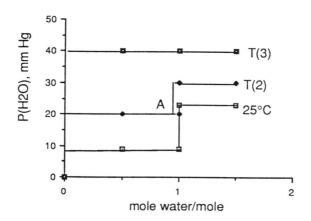

FIGURE 12.6. *Single salt-pair (monohydrate) vapor pressures as a function of temperature. The line at point A has been drawn slightly to the left for graphical clarity. It occurs at 1 mole of water/mole of solid.*

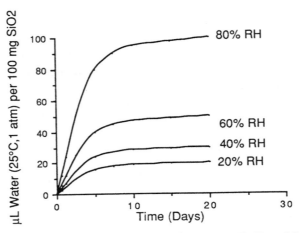

FIGURE 12.7. *Moisture uptake curves for silica at 20, 40, 60, and 80% RH.*

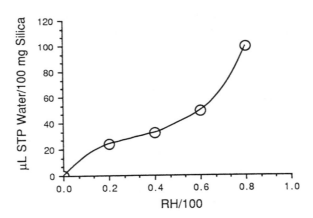

FIGURE 12.8. *The equilibrium levels in Figure 12.7 plotted versus relative humidity.*

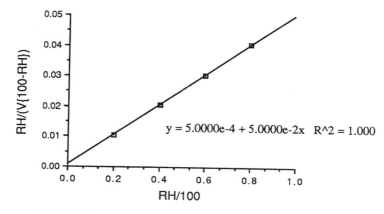

FIGURE 12.9. *Data from Table 12.4 treated by the BET equation.*

second column of Table 12.4. It is customary in isotherm work to convert these adsorbed amounts to the volume that would have been occupied at 0°C and 1 atm, and this can easily be done, e.g., for the first row. The number of moles is $n = 17.5 \times 10^{-3}/18 = 9.75 \times 10^{-4}$ moles. The volume of this at 25°C and 1 atm would be $V = nRT/P = 9.75 \times 10^{-4} \times 82 \times 273/1 = 23.8$ mL. These figures are shown in the third column and are denoted V.

The isotherms of this type are called BET isotherms [3–7]. The data in the third column are shown in Figure 12.8. It can be shown that such data follow the BET equation:

$$RH/[V\{100 - RH\}] = \phi + (1/V_m)[RH/100] \qquad (12.5)$$

Treatment by this equation is shown in Figure 12.9. V_m is here the volume (0°C, 1 atm) of water that just constitutes one layer on the entire surface of

TABLE 12.4 Data from Which Figure 12.9 Was
Constructed, and Conversion to BET Parameters.

RH	mg Adsorbed per 100 mg Silica	V (μL) (0°C, 1 atm)	RH/(V{100 − RH})
20%	19.14	23.8	0.01
40%	26.13	32.5	0.021
60%	39.56	49.2	0.030
80%	79.52	98.9	0.040

the solid sample. RH/[V{100 − RH}] has been calculated in Table 12.4 (last column), and is plotted below versus RH/100. The slope of the line is [$1/V_m$] so

$$[1/V_m] = 0.05, \text{ or } V_m = 20 \text{ mL} \qquad (12.6)$$

This can be converted to moles (n) and then to molecules (N):

$$n_m = PV/RT = 1 \times 20/[82 \times 273] = 8.93 \ 10^{-4} \text{ moles}$$

$$= 6 \times 10^{23} \times 8.93 \times 10^{-4} = 49 \times 10^{19} \text{ molecules} \qquad (12.7)$$

Water molecules in a monolayer will position themselves as shown in Figure 12.10. It is known from other sources that the area occupied by each water molecule is 10 Å^2 = 10×10^{-16} cm^2, so that in this case the entire surface would be the number of molecules times the area of each molecule, i.e.

$$49 \times 10^{19} \times (10 \times 10^{-16}) = 49 \times 10^4 \text{ cm}^2 = 49 \text{ m}^2/100 \text{ mg} = 490 \text{ m}^2/\text{g}$$

Most substances are not "hygroscopic" below 20% RH. Hence if a bag of silica with a surface area of 49 m^2/g or higher is placed in a bottle with a dosage form, then the silica will pick up moisture up to a weight content of 17.5% weight and during this period of the time the dosage form will not (or hardly) pick up any moisture. In general, as a rule, it is said that silica will

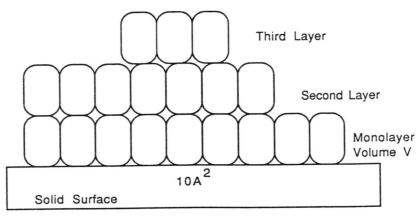

Third Layer

Second Layer

Monolayer
Volume V

10 A^2

Solid Surface

FIGURE 12.10. *Monolayer of water molecules on a solid surface.*

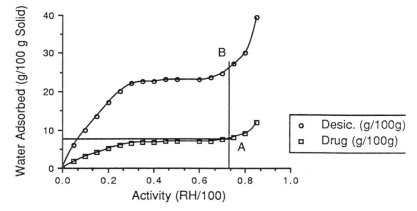

FIGURE 12.11. *Moisture isotherm of silica bag and of a drug product.*

exhaust at 20% moisture. This, of course, depends on the surface area of the silica, and it can be as high as 30%.

Moisture isotherms are of great significance in pharmaceutics. Cases in point are the moisture isotherms of PVP [8] and misoprostol/hydroxypropyl methylcellulose complex [9].

12.5 USE OF DESICCANTS IN PACKAGES

It was mentioned earlier that many products have a critical moisture content (*a* mg/tablet) above which they are no longer stable.

When the drug product is stored in a plastic container, moisture will penetrate, and at a given time, the critical moisture content will be reached (e.g., "A" in Figure 12.11). To prolong the time for this to occur, it is often a practice to include a bag or container of a desiccant, most often a silica bag. Aside from the obvious advantages, there are disadvantages to this as well: cost, appearance, and patient compliance. Bags have often been eaten by misinformed patients. Hence the desiccant should be nontoxic.

Silica (SiO_2) has a very large specific surface area and has a moisture equilibrium curve as shown in curve B in Figure 12.11. In general, it is effective in picking up moisture until it contains 30% water, but this depends on the situation and on the particular sample of silica.

Suppose we have a tablet with an EMC curve of the type shown in Figure 12.11 marked A. At low RH the curve will be almost linear, and the lower portions of the isotherms are shown in Figure 12.12.

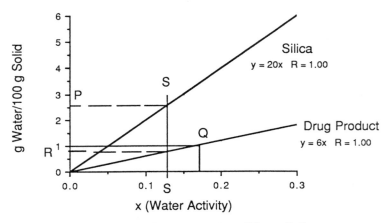

FIGURE 12.12. *Linear portion of Figure 12.11.*

As a dosage form is placed with a silica bag in a bottle, the silica bag will be "dry" and at first it will draw moisture out of the dosage form. This will result in an initial equilibrium where both silica bag and drug dosage form have moisture. This is shown in Figure 12.12 and is best exemplified by example.

Example 12.1

A dosage form has the moisture isotherm shown in Figure 12.12, and is placed in a hermetic (e.g., glass) bottle with a one gram bag of a silica that has the moisture isotherm shown in Figure 12.12 as well. The tablet contains water to the extent of 10 mg of water per one gram of dry dosage form (or 1 gram per 100 g of solid). There are 10 g of tablets (e.g., twenty tablets at 500 mg each) in the bottle, i.e., there is a total of $10 \times 10 = 100$ mg of water in the tablets.

If the silica bag is anhydrous at the time of packaging, how much moisture will leave the dosage form and be adsorbed by the silica originally?

Answer 12.1

In the following, subscript "*si*" will denote silica and "*dr*" drug.

(1) Initial
- silica: 0 mg of water per 1 g of silica
- drug: 100 mg of water per 10 grams of tablets

(2) Moisture isotherms
- silica: $y_{si} = 20\,x_{si}$ or $x_{si} = y_{si}/20$
- drug: $y_{dr} = 6\,x_{dr}$ or $x_{dr} = y_{dr}/6$

(3) Initial equilibrium relative humidities
- silica: $x_{si} = y_{si}/20 = 0/20 = 0$
- drug: $x_{dr} = y_{dr}/6 = 1.0/6 = 0.16$ (point Q in Figure 12.12)

Of course, there cannot be two different relative humidities in the bottle, so after equilibration, m mg of water will have left the drug and have adsorbed on the silica. The amounts of water are, therefore:

- silica: m g water/g silica: $y_{si} = 100m$ (g H_2O/100 g)
- drug: $100 - m$ g water/10 g drug: $y_{dr} = 10(100 - m)$ (g H_2O/100 g)

Note that the total amount of water in the system is $(100 - m) + m = 100$, i.e., unaltered as it should be. The relative humidities are now:

- silica: $x_{si} = y_{si}/20 = 100m/20 = 5m$
- drug: $x_{dr} = y_{dr}/6 = 10(100 - m)/6$

Since at equilibrium the relative humidities are the same, i.e., $x_{dr} = x_{si}$, it follows that

$$5m = 10(100 - m)/6$$

from which

$$30m = 1000 - 10m \quad \text{or} \quad m = 1000/40 = 25 \text{ mg}$$

so

- $y_{dr} = (100 - 25) = 75$ mg/10 g $= 0.75$ g/100 g (point R in Figure 12.12)
- $y_{si} = 25$ mg/1 g $= 2.5$ g/100 g (point P in Figure 12.12)

The relative humidities should be the same (point S in Figure 12.12) as indeed they are:

- $x_{dr} = 0.75/6 = 0.125$
- $x_{si} = 2.5/20 = 0.125$

It would now appear that the silica will always dry out the dosage form, and there could be cases where this would be contraindicated. However, moisture equilibration is not necessarily that rapid [10] and it is only when the silica is more hygroscopic than the dosage form (i.e., initially, a slightly moist silica will dry out at the expense of the dosage form) that this presents a problem.

Example 12.2

A tablet has a critical moisture content of 1.5% (corresponding to an equilibrium RH of 20%) and is produced with a moisture content of 1%. One hundred tablets at 500 mg are packed in a bottle with a 2 g silica bag. The silica bag at an RH of 20% has an equilibrium moisture content of 20%. The bottle allows a moisture penetration of 0.5 mg/day. How long will the product in the package be satisfactory?

Answer 12.2

0.5% of moisture can be picked up before the moisture level is deleterious. The weight of the tablets is 50 g, so that 0.5% of 50 = 250 mg of moisture may be picked up. The silica bag can pick up 20% of 2 g = 400 mg of moisture before it is exhausted. 650 mg of moisture may be picked up, and this will occur in 650/0.5 = 1300 days.

In the above it is assumed that the moisture penetration occurs at constant velocity. This is truly not the case, since as the interior RH increases, the moisture penetration rate will decrease. However, the calculations do not become more refined by introducing this variable, and they do become quite cumbersome.

It should be pointed out that there are other sources of instability than moisture (e.g., oxygen), but from a packaging point of view, moisture is most often the limiting consideration.

It is general practice to assume that the equilibrium moisture curve for dosage forms (mostly mixtures of starch and organic compounds) is of the type shown in Figure 12.11.

12.6 REFERENCES

1. Carstensen, J. T. 1977. *Pharmaceutics of Solids and Solid Dosage Forms*. New York, NY: Wiley, pp. 13–14.

2. Martinez, H., S. R. Byrn and R. R. Pfeiffer. 1990. *Pharm. Res.*, 7:147.

3. Brunauer, S. 1961. *Solid Surfaces and the Gas-Solid Interface*, R. F. Gould, ed., Washington, DC: Am. Chem. Soc., p. 15.

4. Brunauer, S., P. H. Emmett and E. Teller. 1938. *J. Am. Chem. Soc.*, 60:309.

5. Brunauer, S., D. L. Kantro and C. H. Wiese. 1959. *Can. J. Chem.*, 37:714.

6. Carstensen, J. T. 1977. *Pharmaceutics of Solids and Solid Dosage Forms*. New York, NY: Wiley, pp. 68–85.

7. Carstensen, J. T. 1980. *Solid Pharmaceutics, Mechanical Properties and Rate Phenomena*. New York, NY: Academic Press, pp. 46–50.

8. Oksanen, C. A. and G. Zografi. 1990. *Pharm. Res.*, 7:654.

9. Kararli, T. T. and T. Catalano. 1990. *Pharm. Res.*, 7:1186.

10. Carstensen, J. T., T. Y. F. Lai, D. W. Flickner, H. E. Huber and M. A. Zoglio. 1976. *J. Pharm. Sci.*, 65:992.

12.7 PROBLEMS (CHAPTER 12)*

(1) When tablets or capsules are made, they contain different materials with different moisture sorption isotherms. Hence moisture will shift, so that all the powder ingredients in the mixture can be in equilibrium with a *common relative humidity* in the pore space of the particulate system (Figure 12.13).

Since moisture contents frequently are low, the isotherms may often be approximated by linear functions. In this problem the dosage form

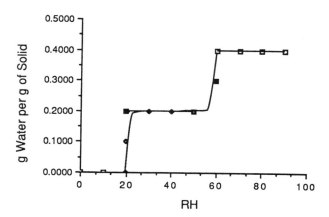

FIGURE 12.13. Stepwise moisture isotherm.

*Answers on pages 244, 245.

is assumed to consist of only drug, D, and excipient, E. Assume that the drug has an isotherm where y_D, the amount of moisture per g of dry drug, depends on the relative humidity, x, by the following equation.

$$y_D = 0.005x$$

and where the equation applying to the moisture content, y_E, of the excipient is:

$$y_E = 0.002x$$

The powder in the dosage form weighs 1.000 g (net) and contains 0.25 g of drug (i.e., 0.75 g of excipient). It contains 100 mg of water per g of dry solid after manufacture.

What is the relative humidity after equilibration of the pore space?

(2) A compound, A, forms a monohydrate, A,aq with a vapor pressure of 12 mm Hg at 25°C (50% RH) and its saturated solution has a vapor pressure of 20 mm Hg at 25°C (83%). The salt pair has a vapor pressure of 40 mm Hg at 40°C and the saturated solution a vapor pressure 48 mm Hg at 40°C. What is the critical temperature for the monohydrate?

CHAPTER 13

Binary Phase Diagrams

Next to the drug itself, a binary system is the simplest pharmaceutical model system. It is of direct importance (1) when drug interacts with moisture, and (2) when it reacts with another excipient in a dosage form (physical or chemical incompatibility).

13.1 PHYSICAL INCOMPATIBILITIES

If two drugs were to be used in a dosage form (e.g., caffeine and methyprylone), then the following behavior is of importance.

Addition of a small amount of caffeine to pure methyprylone will depress the melting point of the latter. For example (Figure 13.1), if $b\%$ of caffeine is added, then the melting point will drop from A to B. Similarly, if a small amount of methyprylone [e.g., $(100 - d)\%$] is added to pure caffeine, then the melting point of caffeine will drop (CD in the curve). Extending this principle, the curves AB and CD will eventually meet (point E) in a simple eutectic point corresponding to the eutectic temperature, T_e, and the eutectic composition X_e. A diagram as shown in Figure 13.1 is called a simple binary diagram. It should be pointed out that the eutectic composition is not a rational molecular ratio of the two compounds (e.g., not one mole of caffeine + one mole of methyprylone), and if it were, then it would be by accident. In fact the two arms of the eutectic diagram ABE and CDE are both Van't Hoff freezing point curves [1–3]. The equation for ABE is:

ABE
$$\ln [m] = -\Delta H_1/R[(1/T) - (1/T_1)]$$
(13.1)

where ΔH_1 is the heat of fusion of compound A, and T_1 is its melting point.

199

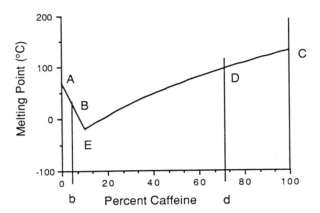

FIGURE 13.1. *Melting point diagram of caffeine (x) and methyprylone (1 − x). Graph constructed from data published by Carstensen [1].*

It is noted that this is of the same type as a solubility curve. Note also that the curve represents liquid with the presence of solid. Similarly, the right leg of the eutectic has the equation:

$$\text{CDE} \qquad \ln[1 - m] = -\Delta H_2/R[(1/T) - (1/T_2)] \qquad (13.2)$$

where the subscript "2" now refers to the compound C. The eutectic temperature is when T from Equation (13.1) equals T from Equation (13.2).

Aside from lyophilization, which will be discussed presently, there are some advantages of eutectics. The so-called PEG preparations are made by melting a drug with polyethylene glycol 2000 or 4000 (PEG, a waxy solid). Upon cooling, the PEG will start congealing first (as fairly large crystals). But when the eutectic composition is reached, both PEG and drug will precipitate out, both in very finely subdivided form (i.e., they will have a large surface area) or precipitate out in an amorphous form. One such product is GRISPEG™ (Herbert Labs, Div. Alergan). In either case (either because of increase in surface area, *A*, or solubility, *S*) the dissolution rate and hence the bioavailability will be improved.

13.2 THE WEIGHT ARM RULE

Consider the eutectic diagram of sucrose and water, shown in Figure 13.2. If one gram of a sugar composition, *e*, is cooled, then it would start precipitating sucrose at point E. As the solution is further cooled, it will continue to precipitate sucrose (and hence become more concentrated in water, i.e., containing relatively less sugar), and if the cooling is stopped at temperature H, then there will be a liquid phase of composition g and solid sucrose. The total amount of material is one gram, and m grams are solid sucrose, $(1 - m)$ grams are solution of composition g. Originally there was one gram of preparation containing e grams of sucrose and $(1 - e)$ grams of water (above point E). Mass balance on the sucrose now gives that

$$m + (1 - m)g = e \tag{13.3}$$

$$(1 - e)m = (e - g)(1 - m) \tag{13.4}$$

The correctness of the latter is best demonstrated by simply multiplying out and showing that the two expressions are identical.

This can be visualized (Figure 13.3) as a weight-arm [1] balanced at point C, with m grams of sucrose suspended at H [length of arm being $(1 - e)$], and $(1 - m)$ grams of solution suspended at G [length of arm being $(e - g)$].

13.3 IMPURITY DETERMINATION

If A is a pure drug substance of melting point T_m, B is an impurity, x denotes mole fraction of the latter, and T_e is the eutectic temperature, then a simple eutectic diagram of the type shown in Figure 13.4 can be created.

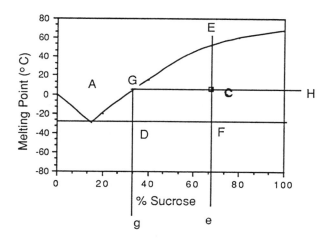

FIGURE 13.2. Eutectic diagram of sucrose.

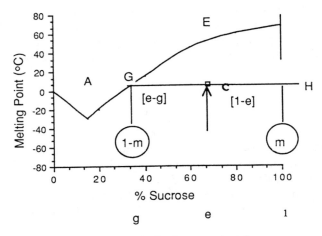

FIGURE 13.3. *Weight-arm principle.*

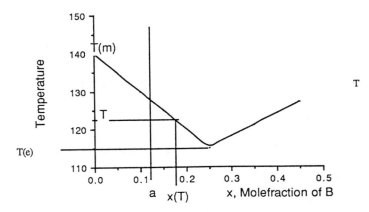

FIGURE 13.4. *Schematic for the Van't Hoff equation.*

202

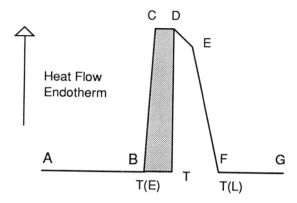

FIGURE 13.5. *DSC trace of substance containing some impurity.*

In differential scanning calorimetry [4], (DSC) the amount of B is most often gauged in the following fashion. As shown in Figure 13.5, a melting endotherm is broken up into n (e.g., $n = 6$) sections, and the area (f) under each determined. The fraction, m, melted at this temperature is the area BCDT divided by the area BDEF (Figure 13.5).

The basis for calculating the amount of impurity, i.e., the fraction, a, of B is the so-called Van't Hoff plotting. The Van't Hoff freezing point depression equation is:

$$x = \Delta H/\{(T_m - T)/(RT_m^2)\} \tag{13.5}$$

The weight-arm rule (applied to the left-hand side of the eutectic diagram in Figure 13.4) gives that $x_T = a/m$.

At any temperature, in DSC, the fraction liquified, m, is equated with x, giving:

$$T = T_m - [RT_m^2 a/\Delta H]\{1/m\} \tag{13.6}$$

So by plotting T versus the inverse of m it is possible to obtain a from the slope. The intercept is T_m and the slope is $RT_m^2 a/\Delta H$.

13.4 COMPOUND SEPARATION IN TABLETS

When both compounds are present and the temperature is above the eutectic temperature, then there will always be some liquid present (i.e., some of the mixture will have "melted"). It is possible to calculate the

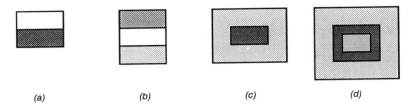

FIGURE 13.6. *Separation methods in tablet design: (a) double layer tablet; (b) triple layer tablet; (c) compression coated tablet; and (d) bicoated tablet.*

amounts of liquid and solid (weight-arm rule) at any given situation. It stands to reason that the eutectic solids will always liquify to some degree if they are in the indicated, triangular areas, and they can therefore frequently not be used as a simple mix in a solid dosage form. This is one reason that some tablets are formulated as "compression coated" tablets (Figure 13.6) or as triple layer tablets. In the former case liquefaction will only occur in the interface between the core and coat, and in the latter case, there will only be liquefaction at contact points between tablets.

There can, of course, also be chemical interaction, which justifies either compression coated tablets or triple layer tablets. Aspirin and dialminate is an example (Bufferin™ is actually a double layer tablet), and a similar reason exists for Dristan™ (which is a triple layer tablet).

13.5 MOLECULAR COMPOUNDS

Some compounds form molecular compounds [5,6] as shown in Figure 13.7. This diagram is essentially a combination of two simple diagrams, and

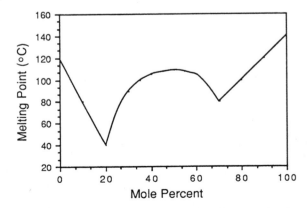

FIGURE 13.7. *Melting point of two compounds that form a molecular compound.*

the point of maximum in the curve always corresponds to a rational molecular ratio of the two components. *dl*-compounds [7] are of this nature (e.g., tocopherol acetate), and hence can have either lower or higher melting points than the optically pure components. Niacinamide and ascorbic acid (both white crystalline powders), if simply mixed and encapsulated, will give rise to capsules where the powder plug will harden (become a "bullet"). The potency is not affected but dissolution for instance, is. The compounds form a 1:1 molecular compound, and what is usually done from a practical point of view is to react them prior to encapsulation (by adding a small amount of ethanol during the blending step). This gives rise to a yellow cake-like material, which can be dried and milled. The powder is then encapsulated and, of course, will now not react further. In water and gastric juice the molecular compound behaves like a weak complex and it dissociates into ascorbic acid and niacinamide. Another example of pharmaceutical interest is Cafergot™ (Sandoz) a combination of ergotamine and caffeine, which gives a complex with enhanced absorption.

13.6 LYOPHILIZATION

It is often desirable to market a drug in the form of a solution. Parenteral dosage forms are one example of this, and syrups and elixirs are another.

Many active drugs hydrolyze in aqueous solution. In solution dosage forms, it is one of the tasks of formulators to find the optimum pH and solvent properties to formulate a product that exhibits the minimum decomposition rate. This should be to such a small extent that the product can be kept at room temperature for, e.g., three years and lose no more than 2–5% of its potency. If the degradation products are harmless, then the product can be marketed as a solution. A product always will have a lower specification limit. Sometimes the drug is so prone to hydrolysis that it is not possible to keep it for any prolonged time in solution. As an example, there are cephalosporins (denoted A below) which hydrolyze rapidly:

$$A + H_2O \rightarrow \text{decomposition products} \qquad (13.7)$$

The stability data of a 10% solution are shown in Table 13.1.

The decomposition is first order, i.e.

$$\ln (C/C_o) = - kt \qquad (13.8)$$

and it is seen from the data in the table that $k = 0.11$ days^{-1}. It is obvious that the product could not be marketed as such, because most of the strength would have been lost at the time it was packaged.

TABLE 13.1 Kinetics of a 10% Aqueous Solution of a Cephalosporin.

Day	mg/cc (25°C)	ln (C/C_o)
0	100	0
2	80	−0.22
4	64	−0.44
6	52	−0.66
8	41	−0.88

There is a technical way of handling this problem. The 10% solution is prepared and filled aseptically as rapidly as possible, for instance over a period of four hours. The vials are then placed in a vacuum oven with cooling capacity (a lyophilizer or freeze drier). The solutions in the vials are frozen and the ice sublimed off at high vacuum. Once the ice (water) is gone, the vials are plugged (by a special method, inside the vacuum chamber) and a sterile cake now exists inside the vial. The product can be reconstituted with water (or other diluent) just prior to use. The cake itself is most often quite stable, so that in this manner the instability has been circumvented to the extent shown below. The product (vial) is then reconstituted just prior to use.

It is seen from Figure 13.8 that as a 10% solution is cooled down from 25°C, it will start "freezing" where line AB cuts the melting curve. What precipitates out at this point are fairly coarse ice crystals. As cooling proceeds this will continue until the eutectic temperature is reached (T_e). Further cooling will then freeze out a mixture (in the eutectic ratio) of very fine crystals of drug and ice. Hence the frozen material will look as shown in

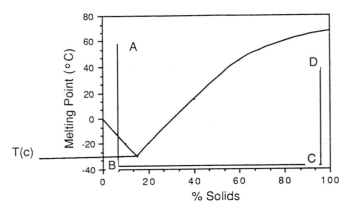

FIGURE 13.8. Lyophilization melting point diagram.

Figure 13.9. It is noted that on sublimation, it is the fine ice crystals that will disappear first since they have a larger specific surface area (area per gram of solid).

In the purest sense of the lyophilization concept, vacuum drying should be carried out until all the water has sublimed off. Then the system will have reverted back to a one-component system with just one melting point. This complete drying is difficult to carry out in practice, so the vacuum is maintained until almost all the water is gone. If the cake were dried to a point where $(100 - b)\%$ of moisture was still present, then on subsequent heating (up to room temperature), some liquid would appear. The amount of liquid would be the higher, the smaller, b [i.e., the higher the percent of water, $(100 - b)\%$, was]. If the amount of liquid (of eutectic composition) is sufficiently large it will rupture the porous cake, and it would "melt back" and form a compact cake that is difficult to dissolve. Melt backs are rejects and should not be used.

At a particular (small) moisture content, $(100 - a)\%$, the amount of liquid will be so small that the cake will be able to support it physically. a is usually about 0.25–0.5%. Hence, in practice, sublimation is carried out until this point is reached. The oven temperature is then raised to 25°C and evacuation continued until the cake is anhydrous.

Melt backs can occur for other reasons as well. Since water's vapor pressure is 0.1 mm Hg at -40°C and 0.28 mm Hg at -30°C, the sublimation is 2.8 times as fast at -30 as at -40°C. It is therefore advantageous to carry out the sublimation as close to the eutectic temperature as possible. Since there are fluctuations in oven temperature from spot to spot, holding the temperature at, e.g., -30°C when the eutectic temperature is, e.g., -29°C, is theoretically satisfactory, but some spots in the oven may then have temperatures above -29°C and produce defects. Such defects can be removed by inspection.

To the present day, lyophilization offers an approach [8,9] for marketing a product whose solutions are not sufficiently stable for marketing as such.

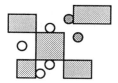

FIGURE 13.9. *State of matter during the freezing cycle. Shaded area is ice. Non-shaded area is drug. Ice is present as coarse crystals and as fine crystals (the latter crystallized below the eutectic temperature). Drug particles are simply crystallized below the eutectic temperature.*

Sometimes (in fact, often) the eutectic will not solidify as a crystalline solid [10], but rather as a glass (an amorphous form). In such cases, the temperature at which total solidification occurs is lower, and is denoted the collapse temperature $T(c)$. The principles above hold in similar fashion for such systems.

It should finally be mentioned that it is possible to produce a powder that is sterile and free of lint and foreign matter. In such cases the powder can be filled aseptically into sterile vials. Reconstitution of powders is not nearly as fast as reconstitution of lyophilized powders.

As a last remark, it is worthwhile to examine the data in Table 13.1 and ascertain that, e.g., four hours of production time does not cause undue decomposition. Four hours is one-sixth of a day, so that the percent not decomposed is calculated from:

$$\ln [C/C_o] = -0.11 \times (1/6) = -0.018$$

from which

$$[C/C_o] = 0.98 = 98\%$$

Hence a 2% excess would cover the loss in production. Product inserts should give information regarding this. If not, such information should be requested from the company. A nurse, for instance, could reconstitute vials in the morning for use in the afternoon (for practical reasons). But this might be a poor practice if solution stability were adverse to such long storage.

13.7 REFERENCES

1. Carstensen, J. T. 1977. *Pharmaceutics of Solids and Solid Dosage Forms*. New York, NY: Wiley, pp. 18–26.
2. DeLuca, P. and L. Lachman. 1965. *J. Pharm. Sci.*, 54:617.
3. DeLuca, P., L. Lachman and H. G. Schroeder. 1973. *J. Pharm. Sci.*, 62:1320.
4. Guillory, J., S. Huang and J. Lach. 1969. *J. Pharm. Sci.*, 58:301.
5. Goldberg, A. H., M. Gibaldi and J. L. Kanig. 1965. *J. Pharm. Sci.*, 54:1145.
6. Carstensen, J. T. and S. Anik. 1976. *J. Pharm. Sci.*, 65:158.
7. Schmidt, W. F., W. Porter and J. T. Carstensen. 1988. *Pharm. Res.*, 5:391.
8. Arakawa, T., Y. Kita and J. F. Carpenter. 1991. *Pharm. Res.*, 3:285.
9. Pikal, M. J., K. M. Dellerman, M. L. Roy and R. M. Riggin. 1991. *Pharm. Res.*, 3:427.
10. Carstensen, J. T. and K. Van Scoik. 1990. *Pharm. Res.*, 25:1278.

13.8 PROBLEMS (CHAPTER 13)*

(1) Two compounds, A and B, form a simple eutectic. The actual melting point depression curve for A has the equation:

$$\ln [1 - x] = - (\Delta H_A/R)[\{1/T\} - \{1/T_A\}] \qquad (13.9)$$

where x is mole fraction of B, ΔH_A is heat of fusion of A, and T_A is the melting point of A. Derive an expression for the "right-hand side" part of the eutectic diagram (e.g., as presented in Figure 13.1).

(2) How is the eutectic temperature (and composition) calculated from these equations?

CHAPTER 14

Micromeritics

14.1 IMPORTANCE OF SURFACE AREAS

It has been mentioned on several occasions that the surface areas of drugs are of importance. In a direct sense, activated carbon [1–4] is used pharmaceutically for its adsorptive properties, and as such is a good adsorbent both due to the force it exerts on external molecules as well as its large surface area. Silica can, as mentioned earlier, be used for desiccation purposes for pharmaceuticals in bottles [5] but can have an adverse effect in certain instances, e.g., when it is used as a filter, where it at times adsorbs proteins [6].

In general, in pharmaceutics, large surface areas are desirable for the purpose of dissolution, but too small particles interfere with operations. Usually the surface area is increased by milling the solid, by precipitating it out finely in the recrystallization step, or by making a PEG melt.

The name "micromeritics" covers the fields of (1) surface areas, (2) particle sizes and their distributions, (3) the nature of the solid surface, and (4) particle shapes.

14.2 SURFACE AREAS

The total surface of a drug is a function of the amount of drug in question. It is, therefore, common to refer to specific surface area, which is the surface area per g of solid. Although such methods as gas chromatography [7] have been reported for the purpose of area (adsorption isotherm) measurement, the most common means of directly measuring surface areas is by gas adsorption. There are forces between molecules in surfaces in con-

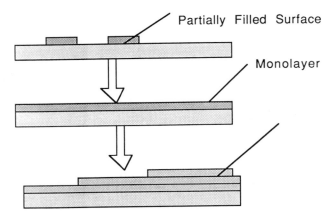

FIGURE 14.1. Nitrogen molecule on a plane surface.

tact with other molecules. These can be molecules in other solids, as seen in compression. In fact, forces between mica plates can be measured directly [8].

As shown in Figure 14.1, when a gas molecule adsorbs onto a solid surface, it will occupy a certain area. In the case of nitrogen, the area is $16\ A^2$ or 16×10^{-16} cm^2.

The measurement is (schematically) done as exemplified in Figure 14.2.

14.3 BET ISOTHERMS

Data of the kind shown in Table 14.1 can be used to calculate surface areas. In such work, nitrogen is used, and the experiment is carried out at

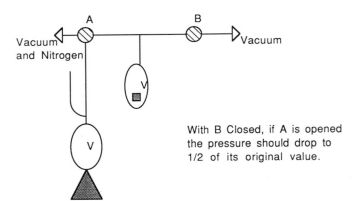

FIGURE 14.2. Schematic of nitrogen adsorption principle.

TABLE 14.1 Equilibrium Absorption Levels from a Nitrogen Adsorption Experiment.

P/P*	v (ml) STP	a/(v{1 − a})
0.2	23.81	0.01
0.4	32.52	0.021
0.6	49.18	0.030
0.8	98.77	0.040

−95°C (the boiling point of nitrogen). Reference is made to the setup shown in Figure 14.2. Valve A is closed, and the McLeod gauge is evacuated. Then a given volume of gas is introduced. Bulb #2 containing the solid is evacuated and valve B is closed. When the valve, A, connecting bulb #1 with bulb #2 is opened, the pressure should drop to one-half of what it originally was in bulb #1, since the two volumes are equal. However, there is a slight negative deviation, ΔP, because some of the gas is adsorbed onto the solid. The amount of nitrogen adsorbed will show up as a loss in pressure (ΔP) at the volume $(2V)$ of the bulbs. This can be converted to number of moles, $\Delta PV/RT$ which in turn can be expressed as volume of gas at 1 atm and 0°C (v ml). The results could be as the ones shown in Table 14.1. The volumes and pressures are converted to the parameter $Y = P/[v\{1 − P\}]$ which is then plotted versus $a = P/P^*$, where P^* is saturation pressure of nitrogen. (At liquid nitrogen temperature $P^* = 1$.)

The so-called BET (Brunauer-Emmett-Teller) equation states that:

$$a/[v(1 − a)] = [1/(v^*c)] + [(c − 1)/(v^*c)]a \approx a/v^* \quad (14.1)$$

the approximation holding when the constant $c \gg 1$ so that, in most cases, the inverse of this slope is the volume of nitrogen, v^*, which constitutes a monolayer. (Note that this number cannot be determined directly, but must be calculated from the slope as mentioned.)

The data are plotted in Figure 14.3, and in the case shown $1/v^* = 0.05$, so $v^* = 20$ mL $= 0.02$ liters, which equals $0.02/22.4$ moles $= 0.00089$ moles, which equals $0.00089 \times 6 \times 10^{23} = 5.4 \times 10^{20}$ molecules. Each of these occupies a surface space of $16 \ A^2 = 16 \times 10^{-16}$ cm², so that the surface of the solid is $5.4 \times 10^{20} \times 16 \times 10^{-16} = 85.7 \ 10^4$ cm² $= 85.7$ m².

If, in a particular instance, the number of molecules in the monolayer is 5×10^{20} then the surface of the solid is $5 \times 10^{20} \times 16 \times 10^{-16} = 80 \times 10^4$ cm² or 80 m². If the sample that had been tested weighed 5 g, then the specific surface area would be 16 m²/g. Some crystalline materials are agglomerates of crystals (see Figure 14.4), and nitrogen adsorption will

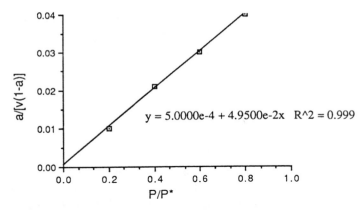

FIGURE 14.3. *Plot of data from Table 14.1, via the BET equation.*

allow measurement of the entire surface, including the crevices (pores). Granules are often porous.

14.4 PERMEAMETRY

Surface areas can also be measured by permeametry. A schematic setup is shown in Figure 14.5. A stream of air enters the bottom of the column, and the resistance that the column of powder offers the air stream is a function of how loosely it is packed (the bed porosity) and of the (external) surface area.

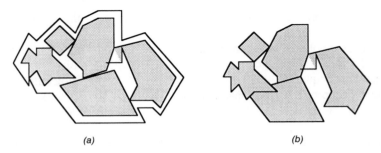

(a)   (b)

FIGURE 14.4. *External versus total surface area of a porous solid. (a) External surface area shown by the continuous contour, (b) internal surface area accounts for internal planes as well.*

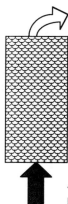

Air Out, Lower
Pressure Drop
is a Function
of Porosity of Bed
and Surface Area

Air enters at higher
pressure than it exits
at

FIGURE 14.5. *Principle of permeation method for measuring external surface area.*

14.5 PARTICLE SIZE DISTRIBUTION

Samples of powders where all the particles are the same size, so-called monodisperse powders, are rare. Only such natural samples as ragweed pollen have sufficiently narrow particle size distribution to be classified as monodisperse. When particle sizes differ within a sample, then the powder is denoted polydisperse. The particle size measurement techniques to be described determine particle size distributions, and the surface area is calculated from the size distribution. Calculating a surface area from length dimensions and assuming the surface to be smooth gives the geometric surface area.

14.6 MICROSCOPY

If a sample of powder is examined under the microscope, a picture as shown in Figure 14.6 may result. There is one particle at 10 μm, two at 5 μm, and four at 2 μm. These data are shown in Table 14.2.

To get the average particle size, it is natural to obtain this as:

$$d_n = (2 + 2 + 2 + 2 + 5 + 5 + 10)/(4 + 2 + 1)$$

$$= [(4 \times 2) + (2 \times 1) + (1 \times 10)]/(4 + 2 + 1)$$

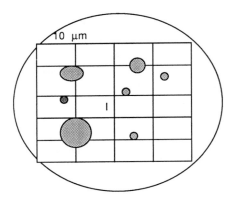

FIGURE 14.6. *Microscopic appearance of data in Table 14.2.*

A more general formula for this is:

$$d_n = [\Sigma nd/(\Sigma n)] \tag{14.2}$$

and this is denoted the arithmetic mean diameter. The general calculation is shown in the first three columns of Table 14.2, i.e.

$$d_n = 28/7 = 4 \ \mu m \tag{14.3}$$

14.7 SURFACE VOLUME MEAN DIAMETER

It should be noted that the volume of a sphere is $V = \pi d^3/6$ and the surface area of a sphere is $A = \pi d^2$, so that the ratio of the two is:

$$V/A = d/6 \text{ or } d_{sv} = 6V/A \tag{14.4}$$

This is denoted the surface-volume mean diameter. In a situation as shown in Table 14.2, the total surface area is

$$A = \pi \cdot \Sigma nd^2 \tag{14.5}$$

and the total volume is

$$V = (\pi/6) \cdot \Sigma nd^3 \tag{14.6}$$

so that the expression for the surface-volume mean diameter would be

$$d_{sv} = 6V/A = \Sigma nd^3/\Sigma nd^2 \tag{14.7}$$

TABLE 14.2 Microscopic Particle Count.

Number of Particles, n	Diameter d	nd	nd^2	nd^3	nd^4
4	2	8	16	32	64
2	5	10	50	250	1250
1	10	10	100	1000	10,000
Totals	17	28	166	1282	11,314

The surface volume mean diameter is different from the arithmetic mean diameter, d_n, as demonstrated in Table 14.2. It is:

$$d_{sv} = 1282/166 = 7.7 \ \mu m \qquad (14.8)$$

as opposed to the value (4 μm) for the arithmetic mean diameter.

It is noticed that in both Equations (14.7) and (14.2) the power of the numerator is one larger than in the denominator (as it should be, so that the unit will be in length). They are referred to as first and third moment diameters (referring to the power of the numerator) respectively.

Another diameter that will be used later is the fourth moment diameter given by:

$$d_{vm} = \Sigma nd^4/\Sigma nd^3 \qquad (14.9)$$

14.8 SIEVING

A means of obtaining particle size distributions is by microscopy. This method is used when particles are fairly small. For coarser particles (50 μm and up), it is more common in pharmaceutics to employ sieving. A sieve is a metal mesh with a defined opening (Figure 14.7).

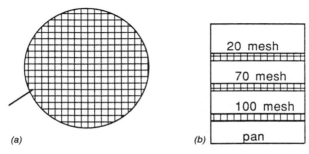

FIGURE 14.7. *Sieve test schematic. (a) Mesh in sieve, (b) nest of sieves.*

The size of the opening is given as a U.S. mesh number which indicates the number of wires per inch. Since the wires have a certain thickness, it is not possible to calculate exactly the size of the opening, but it is necessary to consult a table, such as Table 14.3 (An approximation formula mentioned earlier assumes that the wire has the same width as the opening.)

If a powder is placed on a sieve, then the finer particles will pass through, the coarse stay. In this manner, a sieve will partition a powder sample in two fractions, one that is finer and one that is coarser than the given sieve.

The sieve is constructed so that the bottom of one sieve will fit into the top of another sieve. In this manner it is possible to stack sieves one on top of the other and form a nest of sieves (Figure 14.7). The finer sieves are placed below the coarser ones and they are then shaken. The powder then partitions into a series of fractions, each of which will have particle sizes defined by the confining sieves.

14.9 AVERAGE PARTICLE SIZE BY SIEVING

Suppose 100 g of material is subjected to a sieve analysis and the results in Table 14.4 are obtained.

One method of representing the data would be to report an average particle size or particle diameter. This is done in the following fashion. The first fraction (mesh cut) is finer than 8 and coarser than 10, and constitutes the so-called 8/10 mesh cut. The opening of the 8 mesh sieve is 2400 μm, that of the 10 mesh sieve is 2000 μm, hence the average size is 2200 μm. Similarly the average particle sizes of the other mesh cuts will be as shown in column 4 of Table 14.4.

To obtain an average diameter (the weight mean or mean volume di-

TABLE 14.3 U.S. Mesh Openings.

Mesh No.	μm Opening	Mesh No.	μm Opening
2	9520	60	250
3.5	5660	70	210
4	4760	80	177
8	2380	100	149
10	2000	120	125
20	840	200	74
30	595	230	63
40	420	270	53
50	297	325	44
		400	37

TABLE 14.4 Results from a Sieve Analysis.

Mesh Number	Diameter d (μm)	grams, g on Screen	Avg. d	g × d	4 × Wt/d*
8	2400	0			
10	2000	2	2200	4400	36
20	840	20	1420	28,400	563
40	420	32	630	20,160	2032
100	149	41	285	11,685	5754
Pan	0	5	75	375	2666
*ϱ = 1.5 g/cm³, so 6/ϱ = 4				65,020	11,051

Average diameter d_{vm} = 65,020/100 = 650 μm.
Geometric surface area = 11,051/100 = 111 cm²/g.
Column 5, e.g., 32 × 630 = 20,160 (line 4).
Column 6, e.g., 4 × 2/0.22 = 36 (line 2).

ameter), the weighted average is obtained as shown in the fifth column of Table 14.4, e.g., the first entry is 2 × 2200 = 4400 and so on. The average diameter is therefore the total of these figures divided by the weight, 100, i.e., 65020/100 = 650 μm. This is the fourth moment diameter, as shown below. The formula for d_{vm}, the weight mean diameter, is given by

$$d_{vm} = \Sigma wd/\Sigma w \qquad (14.10)$$

where w is the weight of the fraction that has a diameter d. The weight of the powder on a sieve is the number of particles, n, on the screen, multiplied by the mass, m, of each particle. The mass of a particle of diameter d is its volume times its density, D. The volume is $(\pi/6) \cdot d^3$ so the weight is given by:

$$w = n \cdot (\pi/6) \cdot d^3 \cdot D \qquad (14.11)$$

Introducing this into Equation (14.10) gives

$$d_{vm} = \Sigma wd/\Sigma w = \{\Sigma n \cdot (\pi/6) \cdot d^4 \cdot D\}/[\Sigma n \cdot (\pi/6) \cdot d^3 \cdot D]$$

$$= \{\Sigma n \cdot d^4\}/[\Sigma n \cdot d^3] \qquad (14.12)$$

i.e., the fourth moment diameter. It will hence differ from both the arithmetic mean diameter and the surface volume mean diameter. As the moment goes up, so does the value of the average diameter.

14.10 SURFACE AREA BY SIEVING

It is always possible to obtain an estimate of the surface area of a powder sample from its particle size distribution. In such a computation it is assumed that all the particles have some sort of geometrical form (e.g., that they are spherical) and that they are smooth. The surface area obtained is therefore called a geometric surface area. In the following, this is demonstrated by example, where it is assumed that the true density of the solid is $\varrho = 1.5$ g/cm^3.

Considering, for instance, the 10/20 mesh[21] cut in Table 14.4, the average diameter of the particles there is 1420 μm $= 0.142$ cm. The amount is 20 g.

The first question to ask is: How many particles are there in the mesh cut? The volume of one particle is $\pi \cdot d^3/6$ and it weighs this amount multiplied by ϱ g/cm^3, i.e., the mass of one particle is

$$\varrho \cdot \pi \cdot d^3/6 \qquad (14.13)$$

If there are n particles in the mesh cut, and the weight of the powder on the sieve is W, then

$$n \cdot \varrho \cdot \pi \cdot d^3/6 = W \qquad (14.14)$$

i.e.

$$n = 6W/(\varrho \cdot \pi \cdot d^3)$$

Each particle has a surface area of $\pi \cdot d^2$, so that the surface area, $\underline{a}$, of the powder on the sieve is $n\pi \cdot d^2$, i.e.

$$\underline{a} = n \cdot \pi \cdot d^2 = (6 \cdot W/(\varrho \cdot \pi \cdot d^3)] \cdot (\pi d^2) = (6W/\varrho) \cdot (1/d) \qquad (14.15)$$

The total surface area, A, is the sum of the surface areas from each screen, i.e.

$$A = (6/\varrho) \cdot \Sigma(W/d) \qquad (14.16)$$

The calculation is carried out in this fashion in Table 14.4, and it is seen that the geometric surface area of the 100 g of powder sieved is

$$A = 11,051/100 = 110 \text{ cm}^2/\text{g}$$

The geometric surface area is always smaller than the real surface area.

---

[21] 10/20 implies through 10 and on 20 mesh.

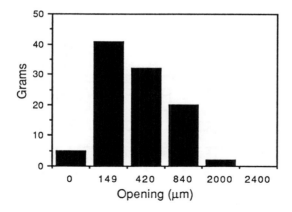

FIGURE 14.8. *Skewed (log normal) particle size distribution.*

14.11 PARTICLE SIZE DISTRIBUTIONS IN SIEVING

In general, distributions of natural occurrences are normal (Gaussian). If a histogram is made of the data in Table 14.4, then a figure such as shown in Figure 14.8 will result. Although the intervals are not equal, it is apparent that the curve is skewed toward the heavier end. This type of distribution often occurs for solids.

To test whether a distribution is normal, the most common (and simplest) method is the following. The data in Table 14.4 are treated as shown in Table 14.5. The actual sieve openings are listed (column 2, note that these are not the midpoints of the confining sieves as in Table 14.4). First is listed the total amount passed through the 10 mesh sieve. Since 2% was retained,

TABLE 14.5 Cumulative Data Treatment of Sieve Analysis Data.

Mesh Number	Diameter d (μm)	% Finer than d	ln d	z^*
10	2000	98	7.60	2.055
20	840	78	6.73	0.672
40	420	46	6.04	−0.100
100	149	5	5.00	−1.645
pan	0			

*z denotes the abscissa value in a normal error table (i.e., the column) corresponding to the value in the bottom of the table corresponding to the % finer than d column expressed as fraction. Column 3 is plotted (ordinate) versus column 2 (abscissa) in Figure 14.9, not giving a straight line. Column 3 is plotted (ordinate) versus column 4 (abscissa) in Figure 14.10 giving a straight line.

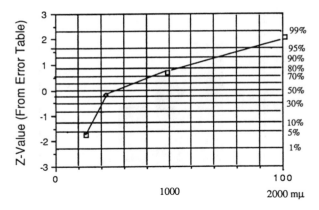

FIGURE 14.9. *Data from Table 14.5 plotted on probability paper.*

98% passed through. Then (in line 2) is listed the total amount that passed the 20 mesh sieve. Since 2% was retained by the 10 mesh and 20% was retained by the 20 mesh it follows that $(100 - 22) = 78\%$ was not retained by the 20 mesh sieve (i.e., 78% of the powder has particles finer than 840 μm).

If the powder particle sizes are normally distributed, then the data should form a straight line, when the cumulative percent (column 3) is plotted on the ordinate of probability paper and the corresponding diameters (column 2) are plotted on the abscissa. It is seen from Figure 14.9 that this is not the case, so the powder is not normally distributed.

Table 14.5 shows the logarithms of the diameters as well. It is seen in Figure 14.10 that when ln d is used as abscissa, then a straight line results,

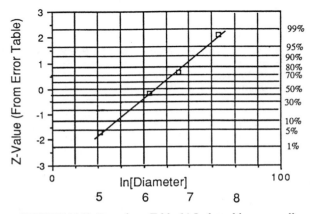

FIGURE 14.10. *Data from Table 14.5 plotted log normally.*

and it is very common that powders are log normally distributed. The reason for this is that when a solid is recrystallized the number distribution will often be close to normal. However, if a number distribution is converted to a weight distribution then the heavier particles are favored. For instance the 10 μm particle in Table 14.2 constitutes 14% by number (1/7) of the particles. The weight is calculated (column 5) as $1282\pi/(6\varrho)$ (where ϱ is the density), and the 10 micron particle in weight percent therefore constitutes $1000/1282 = 78\%$ of the total weight.

14.12 REFERENCES

1. Burke, G. M., D. E. Wurster, V. Buraphacheep, M. J. Berg, P. Veng-Pedersen and D. D. Shottelius. 1991. *Pharm. Res.*, 8:228.
2. Domingo-Garcia, M., T. Fernandez-Morales, F. J. Lopez-Garzon, C. Moneno-Castilla and M. J. Prades-Ramirez. 1990. *J. Coll. and Int. Sci.*, 136:160.
3. Tan, J. S. and P. A. Martic. 1990. *J. Coll. and Int. Sci.*, 136:415.
4. Argawel, R. K. and J. A. Schwartz. 1989. *J. Coll. and Int. Sci.*, 130:137.
5. Ligner, G., A. Vidal, H. Balard and E. Papirer. 1990. *J. Coll. and Int. Sci.*, 136:134.
6. Wahlgreen, M. and T. Arnebrant. 1990. *J. Coll. and Int. Sci.*, 136:259.
7. Long, V. T., B. S. Minkes, T. Matsuura and S. Sourirajan. 1988. *J. Coll. and Int. Sci.*, 125:478.
8. Herman, M. C. and K. D. Papadopoulos. 1990. *J. Coll. and Int. Sci.*, 136:385.

14.13 PROBLEMS (CHAPTER 14)*

(1) Calculate the surface area and the specific surface area of the powder sample in Table 14.2. Assume that the density of the solid is 3 g/cm³.

*Answers on page 246.

CHAPTER 15

Sustained Release Principles

If a drug substance is administered in doses of D at intervals of τ hrs., if the fraction absorbed is F, if the volume of distribution is V, and if the elimination rate constant is k, then the infinite time blood level will be [1]

$$B_\infty = FD/(Vk\tau) \qquad (15.1)$$

Since V, F, and k are givens, it is seen that B_∞ simply becomes a function of the rate, D/τ. Hence, if a dosage form could be developed which would bleed out the drug at this rate, then, if the drug is absorbed throughout the entire GI tract, and with the same absorption rate constant, and if it can be assumed that the transit of the dosage form is with constant velocity, then a sustained release dosage form would be attained.

The picture is very oversimplified, in many respects (but as shall be seen in the following works more or less satisfactorily by many principles). Even in the ideal case shown in Figure 15.1, the blood level curves of a t.i.d. and a one-a-day sustained release preparation of the same drug will not coincide. One might argue that the smoothening of the sustained release would be an advantage, except that it is a rare drug that meets the stated requirements.

If there is a biological window, for instance, then the blood level curve of the sustained release preparation would start decreasing at the time when the window time had been reached, and although the initial rate might be the same, the percent absorbed would be less.

The above assumes that the blood levels are proportional to the dose administered. For some drugs there is a positive displaced dose response curve, and in such a case the sustained release curve could give a higher curve.

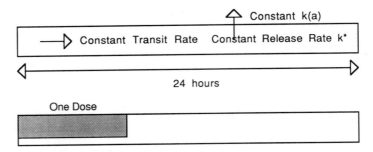

FIGURE 15.1. *Ideal situation for conventional sustained release.*

Since sustained release products are such that one dose replaces many doses, the amount of drug per administration is, of course, higher. For this reason it is necessary both *in vitro* and *in vivo* to assess the danger of dumping, because should a large amount of the dose be accidentally released too early, undesired or even toxic levels could be reached.

The assumption that the absorption rate is constant throughout the GI tract is, of course, unrealistic in most cases (see Figure 15.2).

The principles used in sustained release dosage forms are, in a systematic sense, those elaborated by Fan and Singh [2]; diffusion, chemical erosion, polymer-solvent swelling, and osmotic pumping. Himmelstein [3] comments on Fan and Singh's model, noting that they have:

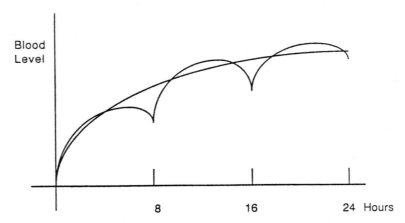

FIGURE 15.2. *Ideal sustained release situation.*

. . . heavy emphasis on mathematical models by arguing that they can be used in the design and development process. Unfortunately, this is not often the case, since most release systems need to be constructed in the laboratory to provide information needed to make the mathematical models work. This suggests that these models are useful for aiding our understanding of delivery systems, but are probably not useful in the preliminary phase of product development with the current state of the art.

It should be pointed out that *in vitro/in vivo* correlations have been, supposedly, worked out theoretically in the case of chlorpheniramine maleate [4]. Because D/τ should be constant, it is desirable that the dosage form be as close to zero order as possible. Even though most of the principles outlined in the following will sustain the release they will most often (except in the case of osmotic pumps) not be linear in time. Modifications [5,6] can, however, be made to linearize non-linear profiles.

15.1 BIOADHESION

It is also a fallacy to assume that the transit rate for the dosage form be constant throughout the GI tract, for it is not. A simple example (Gupta and Robinson, 1991) is that there is a gastric emptying time, so that there is a residence time in the stomach. A residence time is not a constant flow rate, in fact it is exactly the opposite. Further complicating matters is the fact that this emptying time is a function of how much liquid is presented with the dosage form, and the rate of emptying depends on the time after administration.

Several investigators (e.g., Robinson [7–9]) have advocated bioadhesion as a means of attaining better controlled release. By this principle, ideally, the dosage form would affix at a certain spot in the GI tract, and release would take place there. Then the absorption rate constant would certainly be the same, and if the release rate from the adhering dosage form were linear in time, i.e., if D/τ were constant, i.e., if there were zero order release, then, truly, the condition for sustained release would be attained. Ichikawa et al. [10] describe such a system giving zero order release.

Most sustained dosage forms, however, attempt only to achieve a sustained release, and of these, the best would be the ones that attained as linear a release (zero order release) as possible, because of the theoretical restraint that D/τ be constant.

15.2 EROSION TABLETS

The principle of these is depicted in Figure 15.3. Here the active drug is suspended (or dissolved, in the case of oil-soluble drugs) in wax, after which tableting takes place. The tablet contains some disintegrant (usually a surfactant). The wax will flake off (erode) and the flakes will release the active ingredient. The rate of erosion is a function of the amount of surfactant in the wax. An example of this is Ciba's Lontab™ principle. The release takes place by a cube root law, so that it is not quite linear. The rate of release is controlled by the amount of surfactant added.

15.3 COATED BEADLETS

This is the original controlled release principle invented by SKF in the 1950s. A narrow mesh sugar crystal (a so-called nonpareil seed, Figure 15.4) is coated with a suspension (or solution of drug in sugar syrup). This rounded beadlet now contains drug and sugar. It is coated with a mixed film containing both soluble and insoluble material.

The beadlets are coated to a thickness of h. When such a bead is exposed to an aqueous dissolution medium: (1) the water-soluble filler will dissolve and form holes in the film, (2) liquid will penetrate through the pores formed, (3) the liquid will dissolve drug on the inside of the sphere and form a saturated solution, and (4) the drug will diffuse out through the

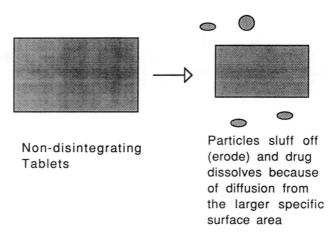

Non-disintegrating Tablets

Particles sluff off (erode) and drug dissolves because of diffusion from the larger specific surface area

FIGURE 15.3. Erosion tablets.

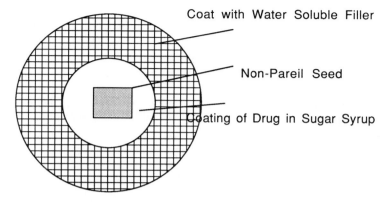

FIGURE 15.4. *Coated beadlet.*

holes. (This principle can also be affected without the water-soluble filler in the film, in which case the liquid will have to diffuse through the film.) The release curve is as shown in Figure 15.5. As long as the solution inside the beadlet is saturated, the release will follow the following relation:

$$\ln [M/M_o] = q(t - t_i) \qquad (15.2)$$

where M is amount not released, q is a constant, and t_i is a lag time as shown in Figure 15.5. q, the slope of the curve, is the smaller and t_i is the longer,

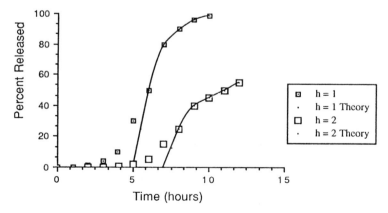

FIGURE 15.5. *Coated beadlet dissolution profile. Two thicknesses are used. It is noted that both the slope and the lag time are affected by the thickness of the coat.*

the thicker the film and the less soluble the filler (the smaller the area of the pores) used in the film. An example of beadlets is Smith Beecham's Contact.

15.4 INSOLUBLE MATRIX

The principle of this is shown in Figure 15.6. A matrix tablet (e.g., methymethacrylate) is made of a water-insoluble material, and the drug is incorporated into this matrix, prior to compression. When it is in contact with liquid, the liquid will penetrate the pores and dissolve the drug, which will then diffuse out. This principle was first described by T. Higuchi (1960). An example of it is the Tral™ tablet (hexocyclium methylsulfate, an anticholinergic). This is marketed by Abbott Labs, and the controlled release principle is called Gradumet™.

This principle was first developed by T. Higuchi [11]. The release occurs by a square root law, i.e., the amount released is proportional to the square root of time, and the full equation is:

$$Q/A = [2DS\epsilon\{L - 0.5S\epsilon\}]^{1/2}t^{1/2} \qquad (15.3)$$

where A is the surface area of the tablet, Q is the amount released at time t, D is diffusion coefficient, S is solubility, ϵ is the porosity of the matrix less the drug, and L is the drug load, i.e., the number of grams of drug per cm³ of matrix. It is noted that for the equation to make sense it is necessary that

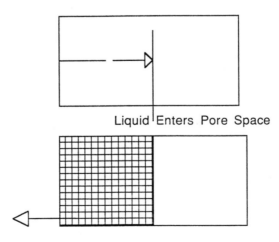

Liquid Enters Pore Space

FIGURE 15.6. *Matrix principle.*

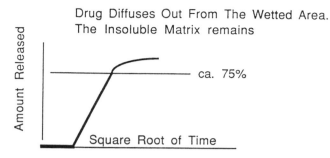

FIGURE 15.7. *Matrix release profile.*

$L > 0.5$ $S\epsilon$. The case where $L < 0.5$ $S\epsilon$ has been solved by Fessi et al. [12]. The release profile is shown in Figure 15.7.

15.5 OSMOTIC PUMP

The principle of this is shown in Figure 15.8. A tablet containing active substance and a controlled amount of somewhat soluble excipient (osmotic excipient), is coated with a material that is water-insoluble, but water-permeable. A pinhole of exact dimensions is then placed in the tablet (by laser). When the tablet comes in contact with water, the water will penetrate into the interior, dissolve drug and the osmotic excipient forms a saturated solution of higher osmotic pressure than the water outside the film. Hence, there will be a constant pressure differential between inside solution and outside dissolution medium, as long as the inside solution is saturated in both osmotic excipient and drug. This pressure will force liquid out of the hole at a constant rate. This gives rise to truly linear (zero order) release.

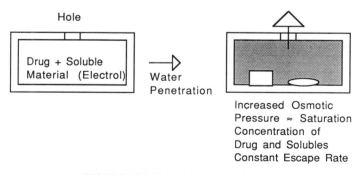

FIGURE 15.8. *Principle of osmotic pump.*

15.6 HYDROGELS

To make hydrogels [13,14], drug is mixed with swellable polymers (e.g., certain molecular weight sodium polyacrylates) and compressed into tablets. When the tablet comes in contact with water, it hydrates and forms a gel, and the drug will have to diffuse out of this gel, giving rise to a sustained action. The release rate is not zero order, but if combined with erosion it may become so. Hydrogels are the type of compound that might be considered for bioadhesives.

15.7 MICROSPHERES

Particularly with advent of protein drugs, microspheres have been used as a sustained release injectable medium, since most proteins have short half-lives. In this type of preparation, an emulsion is made of the drug (protein), in a monomer, and a cross-linking agent is added, so that the outside of the droplet becomes rigid.[22] This is then filtered and washed, and (often) suspended in water, and lyophilized. Sangtvi and Nairn [15] have described the use of ternary diagrams in the design of microencapsulation, to optimize compositions, e.g., of cellulose acetate trimellitate, light mineral oil and solvent (acetone/ethanol). Stjarnkvist et al. [16] have described a series of biodegradable microspheres for this purpose, e.g., polyacryl starch.

15.8 REFERENCES

1. Carstensen, J. T. 1977. *Pharmaceutics of Solids and Solid Dosage Forms.* New York, NY: Wiley, p. 102.
2. Fan, L. T. and S. K. Singh. 1989. *Controlled Release: A Quantitative Treatment.* New York, NY: Springer-Verlag.
3. Himmelstein, K. J. 1991. *J. Pharm. Sci.*, 80:304.
4. Williams, R. L., R. A. Upton, L. Ball, R. L. Braun, E. T. Lin, W. Liang-Gee and L. J. Leeson. 1991. *J. Pharm. Sci.*, 80:22.
5. Scott, D. C. and R. G. Hollenbeck. 1991. *Pharm. Res.*, 8:156.
6. Zoglio, M. A. and J. T. Carstensen. 1985. *Int. J. Pharm. Tech and Prod. Mfg.*, 5:1.
7. Park, H. and J. R. Robinson. 1984. *Int. J. Pharm.*, 19:107.
8. Ch'ng, H. S., H. Park, P. Kelly and J. R. Robinson. 1985. *J. Pharm. Sci.*, 74:406.
9. Park, H. and J. R. Robinson. 1987. *Pharm. Res.*, 4:457.
10. Ichikawa, M., S. Watanabe and Y. Miyake. 1991. *J. Pharm. Sci.*, 80:1062.

[22]Alternatively the protein can be added to a solvent solution of the polymer emulsified in water and dried.

11. Higuchi, T. 1963. *J. Pharm. Sci.*, 52:1145.
12. Fessi, H., J. P. Marty, F. Puisieux and J. T. Carstensen. 1978. *Int. J. Pharm.*, 1:265.
13. Bamba, M., F. Puisieux, J. P. Marty and J. T. Carstensen. 1979. *Int. J. Pharm.*, 2:307.
14. Bamba, M., F. Puisieux, J. P. Marty and J. T. Carstensen. 1980. *Int. J. Pharm.*, 3:87.
15. Sanghvi, S. P. and J. G. Nairn. 1990. *J. Pharm. Sci.*, 80:394.
16. Stjarnkvist, P., L. Degling and Sjoholm. 1991. *J. Pharm. Sci.*, 80:436.

15.9 PROBLEMS (CHAPTER 15)*

(1) A sustained release pellet is used in a product where 20–30% (average 25%) is supposed to release *in vitro* in one hour, and 60–70% is supposed to release in four hours. A batch is made in two portions, A and B, with the following release characteristics:

	A	B
Amount released in 1 hr	15	40
Amount released in 4 hr	50	80

How much A and B should be mixed to make the product conform to specification?

(2) A product is developed as a matrix tablet. Assume that there is no initial lag time, and that 50 mg releases from a 2 cm² tablet in four hours. The fractional load is $L = 0.4$, and the porosity of the dry tablet is 0.1.

How would substituting 20% of the polymer with lactose affect the dissolution pattern?

CHAPTER 1

(1) The integrated dissolution equation for a plate would be:

$$\ln [1 - (C/S)] = -(k'A^*/V)t \qquad (1.22)$$

or

$$\ln [S - C] = \ln [S] - (k'A^*/V)t \qquad (1.23)$$

The data are plotted in the latter fashion in Figure 1.10 (p. 236). It is noted that the intercept is close to $\ln [S] = \ln [100]$ as it should be. It is seen from the slope that $-(k'A^*/V) = -0.00813$, and since $A^* = 1$ and $V = 900$, it follows that $k' = 900 \times 0.00813 = 7.2$ cm/min.

(2) According to Equation (1.21), the rate constant should be larger by a factor of $2^{1/2} = 1.4$.

CHAPTER 2

(1) (a) 71.36   28.5%
     25.1   10.04%
  (b) 0.2066 min^{-1}
  (c) $t = 12.5$ min
  (d) Not equivalent. Would be equivalent if thirty samples were taken during the blending validation.

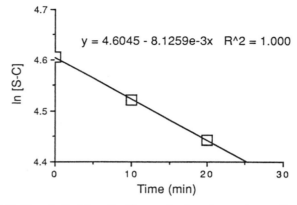

FIGURE 1.10. *Data in Problem (1), Chapter 1, plotted according to Equation (1.23).*

CHAPTER 3

(1) (a) 1.45 g/cm³
   (b) 0.914 g/cm³
   (c) 0.37 (unitless)
   (d) #1 (0.5 cm³)
   (e) 57 mg lactose
   (f) RSD_{final} = 0.05%
   (g) $RSD_{initial}$ = 74.3% RSD_{final} = 0.08%

(2) (a) Fill weight 0.21 × 0.8 = 168 mg

	mg/cap	g/batch
(b) Drug	60	12.48
Mg. stearate	0.84	0.175
Lactose	107.16	22.289
Totals	168	34.944

   (c) Avg wt = 178 mg. Drug content = (178/168) × 60 = 63.6 mg. Fill weight is 100 × (1 − {178/168}) = 6% (<15%) higher than theoretical. Run the machine faster.
   (d) Average fill weight is 200 mg, drug content (200/168) × 60 = 71.4 mg. Fill weight is 100 × (1 − {200/168}) = 19% too high. Reformulate.
   (e) q.s. to 200 mg with lactose. Change magnesium stearate content to 1/2% of 200 = 1 mg:

	mg/cap
Drug	60
Mg. stearate	1
Lactose	139
Totals	200

(f) $x = 0.35 > 0.1$ $(35\% > 10\%)$

(g) 4 min, avg $= 60$, $sd = 29.60574$, $RSD = 49.3429$ $\ln[RSD] = 3.8990$

6 min, avg $= 60$, $sd = 17.82632$, $RSD = 29.71054$ $\ln[RSD] = 3.3915$

$$\ln[RSD] = -0.25375\, t + 4.914$$

(1) Blending rate constant $= 0.25$ min^{-1}
(2) $RSD_o = \exp(4.914) = 136\%$
(3) $x = 60/168 = 0.357$ so $1 - x = 0.643$
     Theoretical $RSD_o = 100 \times [0.357/0.643]^{1/2} = 75$
(4) $\ln[6] = 1.7918 = -0.25375\, t^* + 4.914$
     $t^* = 3.1222/0.25375 = 12.3$ min

(h) The batch used could have a larger particle size (e.g., be from a different manufacturer).

CHAPTER 4

(1) The two energy consumptions are denoted E_1 and E_2. According to Equation (4.4)

$$E_2/E_1 = \ln[500/5]/\ln[500/50] = \ln[100]/\ln[10]$$

$$= 4.605/2.303 = 2$$

(2) Using Equation (4.7), we find that

$$\ln[0.9] = -5q/c, \text{ i.e., } q/c = 0.105/5 = 0.021 \text{ min}^{-1}$$

For the fraction, x_{10}, not milled after 10 minutes we then find that

$$\ln[x_{10}] = -0.021 \times 10 = -0.21$$

so $x = 0.81$, i.e., 81%

CHAPTER 5

(1) (a) The correct answer is 4. The disintegrant should not be granulated, because it is intended for the dissolution or disintegration fluid to penetrate the pore space and interact directly with the disintegrant (crosspovidone), so that it may expand. (Disintegrants add fines to the formulation, and at times it is necessary to include at least some disintegrant before granulation, so there are cases when some of the disintegrant is kept "internal"; it is still fairly active when granulated.) The magnesium stearate should not be covered up with granulation liquid, since it must act directly on the punch walls.

(b) The first three ingredients in the formula add up to 2000 g. The percentages of the first three ingredients amongst themselves are cornstarch $- 100 \times (150/2000) = 7.5\%$, lactose $- 100 \times (1800/2000) = 90\%$ and cornstarch for paste $- 100 \times (50/2000) = 2.5\%$. Aiming, e.g., at a 160 mg tablet weight, an amount x consists of the drug plus the first three ingredients, where x is given by $102.5x = 160$, i.e., $x = 156.1$ mg. 10 mg are drug so 146.1 mg consists of the first three ingredients. The formula per tablet, hence, is:

Drug	10 mg	
Cornstarch 0.075 × 146.1	10.9575 mg	
Lactose 0.9 × 146.1	131.49 mg	
Cornstarch for paste 0.025 × 146.1	3.6525 mg	
Total granulated/dried	156.10 mg	156.1
Crosspovidone 2%	(3.122 mg)	3.12
Magnesium stearate 0.5%	(0.7805 mg)	0.78
Total	160.0025 mg	160.00

It is noted that even carrying out many decimal points, there is still a slight discrepancy in the total, and this is usually adjusted as shown.

300 g makes $300/0.01 = 30,000$ tablets. The above amounts are therefore multiplied by 30 to give the number of grams (rather than mg) of èach of the first four ingredients. This is granulated, dried, weighed, and the two last ingredients are added as a percentage of the weight of the dried granulation.

(c) Add a glidant, e.g., talc (1%), or regranulate to remove fines.

(d) Add more crosspovidone (e.g., an additional 1%).

(e) The formula above with the added talc, and the amount of cross-povidone changed to 3%.

(f) If the material has been regranulated, then, for the next batch to be made, the amount of cornstarch for paste would have to be changed, and the amount of water as well.

(2) The apparent densities are: 2000 kg force: 0.5 g/0.9 cm³ = 0.55 g/cm³. Porosity $\epsilon = 1 - (0.55/1.25) = 0.56$. ln [$\epsilon$] = -0.58; 5000 kg force: 0.5 g/0.5 cm³ = 1 g/cm³. Porosity $\epsilon = 1 - (1/1.25) = 0.2$. ln [$\epsilon$] = -1.61.

Heckel slope: $(1.61 - 0.58)/(5000 - 2000) = 3.4 \times 10^{-4}$ = $1/(3\phi)$; $\phi = 971$ kg force.

(3) If you extrapolate the curves down to the x-axis (Figure 5.23) you get the lag times. You can estimate these to be 2 minutes for the hard shell capsule (t_1), and 6 minutes for the tablet. (This can be done logarithmically as well by plotting ln {amt not dissolved} versus time, and determining where on this line the value ln [100] = 4.605 occurs. This is shown for the tablet below.) The lag time can be calculated from Figure 5.24.

$4.605 = 8.5409 - 0.69315 [t_2]$ so $t_2 = (8.54 - 4.61)/0.693 = 5.67$ min.

The lag time for the hard shell capsule is the wetting time, so that this is 2 min (both for capsule and tablet). Therefore, the penetration and disintegration time for the tablet is $6 - 2 = 4$ minutes.

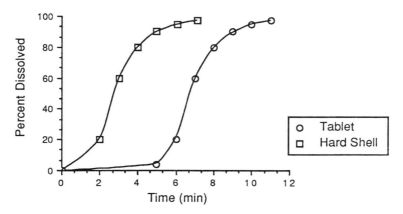

FIGURE 5.23. *Data plotted in Cartesian coordinates.*

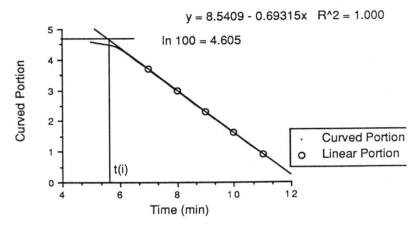

y = 8.5409 - 0.69315x   R^2 = 1.000

ln 100 = 4.605

FIGURE 5.24. *Data plotted as log of remaining versus time.*

CHAPTER 6

(1) $(0.15 \times 7) + (0.2 \times 5) + (0.35 \times 4) + (0.3 \times 0) = 1.05 + 1 + 1.4 + 0 = 3.45\%$

(2) $\ln [(20 - 0)/(40 - 0)] = -k8$ so $k = 0.693/8 = 0.085 \text{ hr}^{-1}$

CHAPTER 7

(1) If the Leeson-Mattocks model holds, then it will.

(2) Not necessarily. That would only be true if there were no bound moisture.

(3) If y denotes loss per year and x denotes moisture content, then

x	1	2
y	1.5	4.5

The equation for this line is:

$$y - 1.5 = [(4.5 - 1.5)/(2 - 1)](x - 1)$$

or

$$y = 3x - 1.5$$

$y = 0$ when $x = 1.5/3 = 0.5$, so 0.5% is the critical moisture content.

(4) The conventional transformations have been made below ($1000/T$ and ln k) and are plotted in Figure 7.19. The rate constant at 25°C ($1000/T = 3.35$) is read graphically to be given by:

$$\ln [k_{25}] = -0.4$$

Using the least squares fit, $\ln [k] = 23.7875 - (7.2188 \times 3.35) = -0.39$.

CHAPTER 8

(1)

Temperature, °C	20	30	40	50	60	70
Solubility, g/100 g water	4	11	32	50	59.5	70
$1000/T$	3.413	3.300	3.195	3.096	3.003	2.914

(a) The plot of solubility data is shown in Figure 8.17. Polymorph I has the lowest solubility at 25°C, so it is the more stable polymorph.
(b) Enantiotropic pair
(c) Heats of solution, H I: $H/1.99 = 9530$ cal/mole
II: $H/1.99 = 1860$ cal/mole
(d) Regardless of form, after 96 hours it is the more stable form that

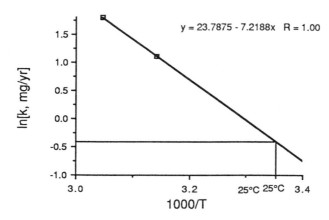

FIGURE 7.19. *Arrhenius plotting for extrapolation. Imprecise method (only two points).*

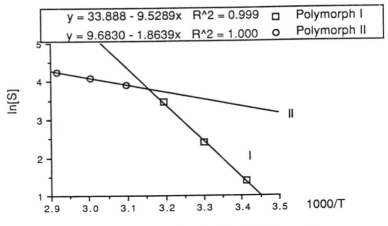

FIGURE 8.17. *Data from Problem (1), Chapter 8.*

will exist in the solid state, and hence it will be form II (which is the more stable at 80°C.

$$\ln [S_{80}] = 9.683 - [1.863 \times 1000/(80 + 273)]$$

$$= 9.683 - 5.278 = 4.405$$

$$[S_{80}] = \exp(4.405) = 81.9 \text{ g}/100 \text{ g water}$$

(e) Yet another polymorph more stable than I ($75 < 81.9$).
(f) Normal processing is at 25°C, so form I should be used.
(g) It can be seen graphically (or calculated) that the solubility of form II is more than that of form I at 37°C, so that II would give as good or better bioavailability, better if the bioavailability is dissolution dictated.

CHAPTER 9

(1) $2d \sin (4) = d \times 2 \times 0.06795 = d \times 0.14 = 1 \times 1.5$, so $d = 10.7$

Note that 8° might be a higher harmonic:

$2d \sin (8) = d \times 2 \times 0.14 = 0.28 \ d = 2 \times 1.5$ also giving $d = 10.7$

The other two angles give different spacings. There can be only three major spacings.

(2) 25°C: $1000/T = 1000/298 = 3.355$

94.90°C: one day $= \ln [0.974] = -0.026344 = -k_{95}/365; k_{95} = 365 \times 0.026344 = 9.616; \ln 9.616 = 2.263; 1000/T = 1000/368 = 2.717$

99.85°C: one day $= \ln [0.96] = -0.0408 = -k_{105}/365; k_{105} = 365 \times 0.0408 = 14.892; \ln 14.892 = 2.701; 1000/T = 1000/373 = 2.681$

Least squares Arrhenius fit of the melt is given by:

$$\ln [k] = 35.32 - 12.2 (1000/T)$$

At 25°C, $1000/T = 3.355$, i.e., $\ln [k]$ should equal -5.611 or $k = 0.00366 \text{ yr}^{-1}$. After three years $-3 \times 0.00366 = -0.0110 = -\ln [C/C_o]$, so the percent retained should be 98.9%, close to that found. Hence the material is in the rubbery state. It should be noted that long extrapolations and assay variances make these conclusions somewhat tenuous.

CHAPTER 10

(1) 80% RH
(2) 71% RH. In 100 g there are 67 g $= 67/90 = 0.74$ moles of urethane, and $33/18 = 1.83$ moles of water, i.e., a total of 2.57 moles. The mole fraction of water is, hence, $1.83/2.57 = 0.71$, i.e., RH $= 71\%$.
(3) Molecular weight of acetone is 58
58 g acetone $= 1$ mole
42 g water $= 2.333$ moles
Total $= 3.333$ moles
Mole fraction of water $= 2.333/3.333 = 0.7 = 70\%$ RH
(0.7) (25) $= 17.5$ Torr is the water vapor pressure, since water's vapor pressure is about 25 mm Hg.

CHAPTER 11

(1) The surface area of bottle consists of that of the two ends $(2\pi d^2/4)$ and that of the side $(h\pi d)$, so for bottle A it would be:

$$(2\pi 5^2/4) + 10\pi 5 = \pi(12.5 + 50) = 196.35$$

For bottle B it would be:

$$2\pi 4^2/4 + 8\pi 4 = \pi(8 + 32) = 125.7$$

The initial moisture penetration rate of bottle B would, therefore, be $(125.7/196.35) \times 0.5 = 0.32$ mg/day.

(2) The USP test assumes that the moisture penetration rate is proportional to the volume of the container and not the surface area. If the principal penetration route is a seal, then this is not an unreasonable assumption.

The volume of a cylinder is $h\pi d^2/4$, so the two volumes would be $10\pi 5^2/4 = 196.35$ cm^3 and $8\pi 4^2/4 = 100.53$ cm^3, i.e., the smaller bottle would have an initial moisture penetration rate of $(100.53/196.35) \times 0.5 = 0.26$ mg/day.

CHAPTER 12

(1) $y = 0.1$. Note that if the dosage form had contained only drug, then the relative humidity would have been $0.1/0.005 = 20\%$ RH and had it all been excipient, then it would have been $0.1/0.002 = 50\%$ RH. The equilibrium relative humidity must lie somewhere in between.

The total moisture is 0.1 g. Of this amount, q grams will go to the (0.25 g of) drug substance and $0.1 - q$ grams will go to the (0.75 g of) excipient. The common relative humidity, x^*, is therefore given by:

$$q/0.25 = 0.005 \, x^* \quad \text{or} \quad q = 0.00125 \, x^*$$

$$(0.1 - q)/0.75 = 0.002 \, x^* \quad \text{or} \quad 0.1 - q = 0.0015 \, x^*$$

Adding these equations gives:

$$0.1 = 0.00275 \, x^* \quad \text{or} \quad x^* = 36.4\% \text{ RH}$$

(2) The vapor pressures follow the Van't Hoff equation and are calculated by converting the pressures ($P_{A,aq}$ for the salt and P_{sat} for the saturated solution) to logarithms and the temperatures to inverse absolute temperatures ($1/T$) and calculating the equations from the lines:

$$\ln [P_{A,aq}] = 27.62 - (7.494(1000/T))$$

and

$$\ln [P_{sat}] = 21.273 - [5.4492(1000/T)]$$

Equating these gives the reciprocal temperature, T^*, at which saturated solution and salt pair have the same vapor pressure, i.e.

$$27.62 - [7.494(1000/T^*)] = 21.273 - [5.4492(1000/T^*)]$$

from which

$$2.0448(1000/T^*) = 6.349 \quad \text{or} \quad 1000/T^* = 3.105$$

$$T^* = 322 \text{ K} = 49°C$$

CHAPTER 13

(1) The percent of "impurity," from the point of view of compound B, would be the amount of A present, i.e., $(1 - x)$. Replacing $(1 - x)$ for x in the equation, and substituting ΔH_B and T_B for the heats of fusion and melting points of B gives:

$$\ln [x] = -(\Delta H_B/R)[\{1/T\} - \{1/T_B\}] \qquad (13.10)$$

(2) The two curves intersect at a common temperature, T_e, the eutectic temperature. So expressing Equations (13.9) and (13.10) in terms of $1/T_e$ gives:

$$1/T_e = -[\ln (x) - (\Delta H_B/R)\{1/T_B\}](R/\Delta H_B) \qquad (13.9A)$$

$$1/T_e = -[\ln (1 - x) - (\Delta H_A/R)\{1/T_B\}](R/\Delta H_A) \qquad (13.10A)$$

Equating these gives

$$[\ln (x) - (\Delta H_B/R)\{1/T_B\}](\Delta H_A) = [\ln (1 - x) - (\Delta H_A/R)\{1/T_B\}](\Delta H_B)$$
$$(13.11)$$

which cannot be solved in closed form.

CHAPTER 14

(1) Note that 1 μm $= 10^{-4}$ cm, 1 μm$^2 = 10^{-8}$ cm^2, and 1 μm$^3 = 10^{-12}$ cm^2. The surface of the particles that are 2 μm large, for example, would be as follows.

The diameter is 2 μm, i.e., 2 $\times$ 10^{-4} cm, so the surface area per sphere is $\pi d^2 = 3.14 \times 4 \times 10^{-8}$ cm^2 ($\pi = 3.14$ used).

There are $n = 4$ particles, so that the surface area of the four particles is 4 $\times$ 3.14 $\times$ 4 $\times$ $10^{-8} = [4 \times 4] \times 3.14 \times 10^{-8} = nd^2 \times 3.14 \times 10^{-8}$.

Hence, the numbers in the fourth column in the table may be multiplied by 3.14 $\times$ 10^{-8} to obtain the surface areas. Thus, the total surface area is this number times the sum, i.e., 166 $\times$ 3.14 $\times$ $10^{-8} = 521 \times 10^{-8}$ cm^2.

To get the *specific* surface area, the total surface area must be divided by the weight (in grams) of the sample. The weight is obtained by the volume $\times$ density.

In the first row the diameter is 2 μm, i.e., 2 $\times$ 10^{-4} cm, so the volume of one sphere is $\pi d^3/6 = 0.52 \times 8 \times 10^{-12}$ cm^2 ($\pi/6 = 0.52$ is used).

There are $n = 4$ particles, so that the volume of the four particles is 4 $\times$ 0.52 $\times$ 8 $\times$ $10^{-8} = [4 \times 8] \times 0.52 \times 10^{-12}$ cm^3. The weight is the density times this figure, i.e., 3 $\times$ [4 $\times$ 8] $\times$ 0.52 $\times$ $10^{-12} = nd^3 \times 1.56 \times 10^{-12}$ g.

Thus, the numbers in the fifth column in the table may be multiplied by 1.56 $\times$ 10^{-12} to obtain the weights. The total weight is this figure times the sum, i.e., 1282 $\times$ 1.56 $\times$ $10^{-12} = 2000 \times 10^{-12}$ g $= 2 \times 10^{-9}$ grams.

The specific surface area, hence, is 521 $\times$ $10^{-8}/(2 \times 10^{-9}) = 2600$ cm^2/g.

CHAPTER 15

(1) The fraction of A is denoted x, and the fraction of B is denoted $(1 - x)$. The one-hour lower criterion demands that:

$$x15 + (1 - x)\,40 = 20 \text{ from which } 25x = 20 \text{ or } x = 0.8$$

The one-hour upper criterion demands that:

$$x15 + (1 - x)\,40 = 30 \text{ from which } 25x = 10 \text{ or } x = 0.4$$

so, as far as the first hour point is concerned, between 40 and 80% of A can be used. The four-hour lower criterion demands that

$$x50 + (1 - x)\, 80 = 60 \text{ from which } 30x = 20 \text{ or } x = 0.67$$

The four-hour upper criterion demands that:

$$x50 + (1 - x)\, 80 = 70 \text{ from which } 30x = 10 \text{ or } x = 0.33$$

so, as far as the four-hour point is concerned, between 33 and 67% of A can be used.

That means that between 40 and 67% of A should be used.

(2) The fraction of lactose (which is soluble) becomes $0.2 \times (1 - 0.4) = 0.12$. L is still 0.4, however, ϵ increases from $(0.1 + 0.4) = 0.5$ to $(0.1 + 0.4 + 0.12) = 0.62$. The other parameters remain unaltered.

249